CHILDREN
PRACTIC

T0229816

CHILDREN IN PRACTICE

BY

JOHN PETERSON

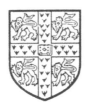

CAMBRIDGE
AT THE UNIVERSITY PRESS
1959

CAMBRIDGE UNIVERSITY PRESS
Cambridge, New York, Melbourne, Madrid, Cape Town,
Singapore, São Paulo, Delhi, Tokyo, Mexico City

Cambridge University Press
The Edinburgh Building, Cambridge CB2 8RU, UK

Published in the United States of America by Cambridge University Press, New York

www.cambridge.org
Information on this title: www.cambridge.org/9781107695238

First published 1959
First paperback edition 2011

A catalogue record for this publication is available from the British Library

ISBN 978-1-107-69523-8 Paperback

CONTENTS

Preface   *page* vii

Introduction   I

   I   PHYSICIAN AND ENVIRONMENT   7

   II   PHYSICIAN AND NEIGHBOURHOOD   21

   III   NEIGHBOURHOOD AND CHILD   29

   IV   NEIGHBOURHOOD, SCHOOL AND HOME   46

   V   DISCIPLINE AND THE CHILD   67

   VI   PHYSICIAN AND CHILD   84

   VII   THE EXCEPTIONAL HOME   107

   VIII   THE INFANT AT HOME   150

   IX   THE CHILD AT SCHOOL   163

   X   THE HANDICAPPED CHILD   192

Index   219

PREFACE

This book is written to assist the medical student to see his child patients within their social context. It aims to describe what he can do for the child within that context and to indicate what others are doing for him.

The drafts have been read at various stages by Dr E. M. Creak, Dr C. F. Harris, Dr E. B. Strauss, Professor R. M. Titmuss and Dr M. Young, all of whom are associated, in one way or another, with activities under this roof. I am very grateful for their help and advice. They have curbed some of my waywardness; but the errors of omission and commission are acknowledged, regretted, and rightly claimed as entirely my own.

JOHN PETERSON

UNIVERSITY HOUSE
BETHNAL GREEN, LONDON, E. 2
July 1958

INTRODUCTION

This book is based upon the experience of teaching medical students during the past ten years. Within a year or so of coming to me they will have embarked upon their professional careers and have begun to assume full responsibility for their patients. As that time comes nearer, they become uncomfortably aware of the personal significance of the dictum that medicine is the most social of studies, and they cast around for some information which will assist them, partly to understand what is going on in the hospital, but mainly to face the new aspect of medicine that awaits them in general practice.

They have already taken a series of orderly steps involving considerable mental and emotional gymnastics, from academic study towards the patient in their own waiting rooms. They have progressed safely from the study of the dogfish and rabbit to the very different study of human anatomy and physiology; from the impersonal limb on the slab to the very different study of the patient in the ward and the theatre. They have gone from the order and cleanliness of the ward to the hubbub of out-patients; and from there they have gone to casualty to see medicine begin with the removal of mud and blood and torn clothes. Midwifery has taken them into people's homes. Will they narrow their field of vision there—and later in their own practices—to the physical facts which are presented to them or will they, as good biologists, widen their vision to see those facts in as large a context as possible?

The whole emphasis of their teaching is upon the necessity of the wider view. Familiar difficulties arise, however, when the student asks for facts. He finds that the experts are many and that they are agreed, only on three things: that there is a paucity of fact, that the application of the known fact is not clear, and that what is done in practice is often demonstrably wrong.

The students come to me when they are in the Children's Department, and the purpose of the course is to get them ready to meet the child in general practice. They are already accustomed to dealing in a workmanlike manner with subjects 'the causes of which are unknown', and it seems to me that the best service that can be rendered to them is to encourage them to enter the field of environmental study in the same workmanlike mood that they bring to other fields. Because I have been there longer, it is helpful to them to watch my attempts at understanding the field and to listen to my speculations about it. The end result cannot be to equip them with new techniques. The object must be, it seems to me, to fire them with curiosity about man and his ways and to encourage them to look around with care as they come to experience the fascination of environmental study.

This book is neither a convenient guide to the social services nor a handbook on bringing up children; neither an anthropological treatise nor an educational discourse. It aims to be a book useful to men and women who have soon to undertake full professional responsibilities towards children. It will have succeeded at least in part if, after reading it, they feel a little more confident in dealing with the child in their own surgery. It will have succeeded wholly if it also fires some to pursue environmental studies. Academic psychology was given new life and meaning by the medically trained; perhaps the same may happen to the other studies of man.

DESIGN

The book is designed with Chapter VI, 'Physician and Child', as its centre. The chapters which precede are preparatory, and deal with the larger notions of environment, aiming to get the physician to the position where he may see the child in perspective within his environmental context. Thereafter, facilities and procedures are recited, together with some of the difficulties in applying them to common problems.

(1) *Physician and environment*

The book begins by defining its province as the sphere of environment which lies between that in which the diseases of the individual patient are presented to and treated by the individual doctor, and that in which the preservation of the public health is achieved by the proved methods of the Medical Officer of Health. Among the difficulties in studying this area are that people, even within the British Isles, live their lives in an enormous variety of ways, and that (partly in consequence of this) doctors and all observers differ enormously in their judgments about these ways of life. The doctor is, however, the only person who can be equipped to see the effect of illness, disease, handicap or accident, upon the life of a child and his family. To do so he must have a sound knowledge of both medicine and neighbourhood, of emotions as well as endocrines.

Consideration is given to the notion of social pressures; the reasons why there is greater awareness of them today, the effect of this upon medical thought, and the difficulties which a professional training may impose in coming to understand the parents' and patients' concept of disease.

(2) *Physician and neighbourhood*

In the second chapter attention is focused on the problem of understanding a neighbourhood, whether urban or rural. The orderly description of a neighbourhood can give some notion of how the individual will go through his life-cycle in that neighbourhood. Thus a basis of comparison is evolved from which the doctor can examine his own assumptions about life there. Human conduct, that is to say, can be understood only within its context—and it is not particularly easy to identify that context. As the grossly economic causes of disease decline in importance, the doctor, if he is to understand what is presented to him, is increasingly compelled to attempt to identify the most difficult group of factors within that context: neither bricks nor micro-organisms, but morals and beliefs, axioms and assumptions. In doing so, he will realise that

3   1-2

reactions and adaptations to events are determined by the way of life, and that the felt needs of people do not necessarily appear to the observer to be either desirable or necessary consequences of the facts as he understands them.

(3) *Neighbourhood and child*

The child is subject to the way of life of his neighbourhood and of his family. In countless ways the child adapts. To clarify the forces to which he must adapt, a distinction is drawn between the objective and subjective factors in a way of life, and folkways, mores, laws and ethical principles are identified. Then, with illustrations from family life, it is shown that demands are made upon groups and individuals; associated with the demands are expectations, and these give rise to assumptions and beliefs. Some of the many pressures which come to bear upon the infant in the home are described.

(4) *Neighbourhood, school and home*

The demands of the neighbourhood and school are necessarily different from those of the home, and each category may be either in harmony or in conflict with the others. Because of the importance given to it in educational practice, and because of the increasing public assumption of its importance, the demand that children must play and not work is examined.

Some of the general pressures which schooling brings to bear are then considered. Educational aims, particularly those of Froebel and Montessori, are outlined and compared with the more traditional outlook. The possibility that any of these outlooks may be in conflict with the way of life of the home is examined, and the relationship of school and family discussed.

(5) *Discipline and the child*

The sanctions which are permitted to ensure the safety of the child and of his society differ in the home, at school, and in the neighbourhood. The distinction between punishment and welfare is pointed out in this chapter. Five characteristics of punishment are enumerated. An attempt is then made to describe punishment in the home, where it is least explicit, at school, and finally at the juvenile court, where it is most explicit and at the same time consciously concerned with welfare.

(6) Physician and child

So far the topic has been the larger environmental problems: the difficulty of understanding social pressures, the possibility of describing them at work in the neighbourhood, of seeing the child growing within them and being compelled to conform. Now attention turns to the child as he is presented to the doctor. Some of the pitfalls and limits in understanding the child are described. These are followed by some illustrations of factors in treatment and an account of the methods of child guidance.

The chapters which follow, 'The Exceptional Home', 'The Infant at Home', 'The Child at School', and 'The Handicapped Child', are more detailed. They describe the facilities available for the remedy of some common problems and indicate some of the difficulties in their application.

(7) The exceptional home

An account is given of the contemporary household, of the immediate and extended families, in order to sketch in the background of the normal home. Then seven types of exceptional homes: (i) the unattached, (ii) the dependent, (iii) the inadequately housed, (iv) the unmarried, (v) the childless, (vi) the disturbed, and (vii) the ineffective, are considered together with the facilities available to assist them.

(8) The infant at home

An account is given of the maternity and child welfare services, of their intention and development, of the use made of them, of current criticism and recent experiments in maintaining infant and child health at home and nursing the sick child there. The relevance of these provisions to the family doctor is considered.

(9) *The child at school*

The chapter begins with a short account of the day nursery and nursery school. It continues with a reference to the parents' obligations and then describes the provision made for schooling and some of the problems which face education authorities. The medical and health services of the schools are then reviewed and some reference made to the relationship between these services and the family doctor.

(10) *The handicapped child*

Reasons for considering all exceptional children together are put forward. The problem of handicapped children is considered mainly in the light of mental handicap. The problem of telling parents is considered, together with their reactions. The objects of management and some of the means by which they may be attained are stated. The same ground is briefly covered in respect of blind and deaf children.

CHAPTER I

PHYSICIAN AND ENVIRONMENT

ENVIRONMENTAL ASPECTS OF MEDICINE

This book is concerned with one aspect of a biological principle: that organisms are interactive with and interdependent upon their environment. It is concerned with environment as it comes to bear upon the child—not with the whole of the environment, but with the interrelation of the child and family, family and neighbourhood, neighbourhood and the general pattern of national life. 'Social Medicine', it has been said, 'is the study of those environmental factors which affect health, and the application of that study to the benefit of man. It has two main applications: (1) The use of this knowledge for the benefit of the individual both in health and in disease:... (2) The use of this knowledge on a community basis.'[1] Here, however, little or no attempt is made to deal with those environmental factors which are ordinarily regarded as public health. The purpose is rather to consider, in relation to children, that sphere of environment which, Lord Horder said, 'lies between that in which the diseases of the individual patient are presented to, and treated by, the individual doctor and the sphere in which the preservation of the public health is achieved by the proved methods of the Medical Officer of Health. This largely untilled field includes all the environmental factors which influence the citizen's health and happiness: his conditions of working, his home life, his sense of security or insecurity, and his ignorance of the things that make for the salvation of his body and his mind.'[2] 'To make Medicine a complete science in the service of man', he says in the same article, 'we must see that it infiltrates the important and now more clearly perceived sphere—as yet largely neglected—of social need.'

It is often convenient, in considering the enormous range of

[1] W. Hobson, *B.M.J.* 2 (1949), 126.
[2] Lord Horder, *B.M.J.* 1 (1949), 557.

7

biological possibility, to regard these environmental aspects as relatively constant. The purpose in this book, on the other hand, is to open up this range of environmental possibility while holding the biological aspects relatively constant. The one process is, of course, as artificial as the other. The intellectual feat is to bring the two processes together, to see the individual child interactive with and interdependent upon his environment. The separation is a mere convenience—to neglect the one, in practice, is as foolish as to neglect the other. Lord Horder, on the occasion quoted above, put his warning thus:

> There has today opened up for the statesman, the sociologist, and the physician a large field for their inquiry and their action, and this field is common ground. The man of Medicine must not spend all his time in this field; he must go apart, whether in the laboratory or at the bedside, or, like Harvey, walk under the trees rapt in thought so that by observation, by experiment, and by contemplation he may keep Medicine dynamic. For it is *through Medicine* that he makes his contribution which no-one else can make. To stand aloof from the work going on in this same field is to do a disservice not only to society but to Medicine itself; but to become entirely absorbed in it is to do a disservice no less serious.
>
> Yes, but the contribution that Medicine makes must be fitted into the social structure of the day—'fitted into', mark you, not just attached.

The purpose, that is to say, is to consider the child as a social creature, who loves his Mum, hates the kids up the road, is afraid of the dark, and is bored by school; who submitted to napkins and woollies, now washes (when supervised) behind his ears and remembers (when Mother is about) not to burp; who has learnt to enjoy lollies and roast beef, tea and the telly; who knows about God Save the Queen, the Archbishop of Canterbury and you mustn't be caught swearing or pulling girls about (but older people are more careless); who has met the doctor, copes with the teachers and avoids the copper. The creature, that is to say, whom parents 'have', neighbours endure and the doctor learns to see not only as an appendage to lacerated hands and knees, as the temporary habitat of the invading germ, but also as a creature about whom

8

mother may be worried: 'He doesn't like school. I can't do anything with him. He has nightmares.'

Two sets of difficulties present themselves: first, that this caricature will not fit some children at all. If the way of life in the British Isles were uniform, if there were no regional differences, no occupational or class differences, if there were one political, philosophical and religious outlook, if everyone were agreed on the way to bring up children, it might be possible to draw acceptable generalised pictures of children which might in turn be serviceable. The facts are, however, plainly otherwise.

Second, and of rather more importance, however, is the difficulty that each one of us sees the different ways of life through his own and individual eyes—the fact that doctors themselves are products of diverse groups, are themselves uniquely made and developed, with differences in outlook and values. Each one of us has his own—and unique—experience of life. This is a matter of primary importance to environmental study.

We accept without difficulty in everyday life that there are individual differences between people: all professions recognise 'opinion'; and differences of opinion which derive from what is peculiar to one man and another in the way of ability and experience. Instruments—thermometers for example—are standardised, more or less accurately, one against the other. Yet in reading instruments some people give different responses from others. Astronomers long ago discovered that the reaction times of individual observers were not identical, that some were regularly quicker, some slower than others; and they learnt to compensate for this more or less constant error by the 'personal equation'.

Another order of difficulty arises, however, when human life is observed. Although it is false, as we come painfully to learn, that emotions never enter the laboratory, when we move out of the laboratory to look at man, it is quite clear that there is a bewildering array of unclassified yardsticks used, with different values inevitably attached to them, and emotion frequently invested in the results of applying them. Whether Muslim or Orthodox, Catholic or Communist, we each according to our lights make our own judgments. The judgments differ not principally because of an ability or inability to perform simple exercises, but because the frames to which the observations are referred are different. Because of our beliefs, our outlooks, we see different things; because of these beliefs and outlooks, when we see the same things, we may place different values upon them. The old joke about the psychiatrists who greet each other every morning by saying, 'Hullo, how am I?', contains an elementary lesson. Each observer is his own psychiatrist and learns about his own frame of reference, his assumptions and beliefs as he comes to investigate those of other people. This is not a dangerous procedure: truth flourishes in light rather than dark places. It is, however, not an easy procedure.

This difficulty must be recognised, for it is the difficulty of everyone interested in man. Manès Sperber has recently put it this way:

The psychologist is implicated in every explanation he gives of Man. His situation before the object of his researches too often resembles that of a guardian whose prisoner has taken him captive. It is the inextricable confusion and promiscuity between subject and object which gives psychology its uncertain character and makes it now a therapeutic technique, now an art or an esoteric discipline, now a sectarian school, a philosophy of life, or a *mystique*. In the realm of physics, differences of opinion reflect differences of experimental knowledge; in interpretative psychology, they express the opposition of two consciousnesses, embodied in two psychologists. In the first case it is the laws of nature which are in question, in the second the psychologists themselves, their pasts and their passions.[1]

SOCIAL PRESSURES

We may begin by saying that we are all subject to social pressures— forces that come to bear upon us, that make us the products of our culture and contribute to make us the persons we are. That this statement may sound both highly artificial and contrary to common sense may be a fact; but neither point constitutes ground for its

[1] In *Encounter*, VI (1956), 6, 66.

absolute rejection. Most of us have long forgotten that the notion that the earth moves round the sun is flatly contrary to the evidence of our senses, and only one in a thousand would know how to begin to demonstrate the notion. We talk of being 'as light as air', 'as free as the air', and we mean what we say. We do not in our daily behaviour accept that there is a physical force pounding down upon us—in spite of an interest in science fiction, in spite of the daily weather forecasts or our pains in flying and penalties in gliding. To demonstrate its existence there have to be difficult journeys to great heights, to great depths, highly artificial experiments and recourse to mathematics.

Factors contributing to awareness of social pressures

It is not surprising that there has arisen an increased social awareness. The reasons may be summarised as follows: (1) We live within a swiftly moving culture; (2) that culture is becoming increasingly complicated and the functions of individuals and groups markedly differentiated by specialisation; (3) the experience and conduct of the war drew attention to social needs and forces; (4) after the war there arose the occasion, during the reconstruction phase, for the provision of 'Welfare', in which the practice of medicine, and consequently medical thought, was much involved; and (5) in this period, with vastly improved communications, culture conflict became obvious.

(1) Change

Cultures rise, decline and then fall; rarely, if ever before, has a culture gone on for nearly two centuries at an ever-increasing rate of change. Just as we do not ordinarily think of ourselves as living pressed down by the atmosphere or moving daily around the earth's axis, we do not in everyday life accept that the way of life changes around us. Nevertheless, the everyday equipment changes. Going back fifty years we find that the child of that time grew into a world without television, radio, telephone, air-transport, effective motor-road transport, dictaphones, duplicators, typewriters, electrical home equipment and many more amenities; that he grew into a world that did not practise social security, that accepted class differences, had not heard of Freud, and that probably believed in progress. Today it may well be true when grown sons and daughters say to their parents, 'You do not understand'. Father may think that he 'moves with the times'; but can it safely be assumed that the older generation do in fact 'keep up with the times'?

(2) *Specialisation*

We live, too, within a highly differentiated culture. Culture depends upon the division of labour, and never before has the degree of division of labour within the professions, for example, been so great and the consequent complication and differentiation been so extreme. Within medicine, can it be assumed that the daily experience of the M.O.H., the G.P., the psychiatrist and the orthopaedic surgeon, to take only larger categories, give each as much common form of thought and feeling as there was between all doctors fifty years ago? There is a whole host of professions, trades, occupations, each giving the individual markedly different experience of life.

(3) *The war*

British public assumptions about man's behaviour were undermined as a result of personal experience during the last war. The realisation that civilised man could torture, starve, bomb, exterminate in the mass, undermined, if it did not destroy, many assumptions about the goodness of man. The need to maintain and improve the morale of both civilians and service personnel, the need to attack the morale of the enemy by way of propaganda, and the desire to use the human material available as carefully and as effectively as possible, turned conscious attention to social needs and forces. Furthermore, during the course of the war, the assumption grew that many of our human ills were attributable to social causes, and that they were remediable by social action. After the war, as the new social services came into operation, it was found that the problems needing solution had shifted from the gross and economic to the individual and social; public assistance, for example, was a relatively crude system of standardised payments; post-war National Assistance has come to see the need of the old lady to keep her budgie.

(4) *Change in medical thought*

The National Health Service Act brought new emphasis in medical thinking and teaching. J. Rickman, writing of medical education, summarised the view at that time:

There are two ways in which a doctor can get instruction. He can be taken by his teacher into the patient's environment and be told there what factors have led to the ailment, what difficulties lie in the way of the remedy, and what chances there are, all things taken into consideration, of recovery. The teacher and his pupil make an entry into the patient's life, they enter his region of 'social space', and do what they can to bring some easement within it. The apprenticeship was an example of this kind of medical education. The second, the more modern way, is different: the patient is drawn into a region where he is isolated from usual social contacts and interests, and is examined by a number of hospital departments which have specialised on one or other aspect of the mechanism of his body or mind. The criterion on which the laboratory departments report is basically a statistical one: the findings lie within the normal limits for the age group of the patient examined.

Contrasting these two generalised methods of instruction and calling the former 'individual or apprenticeship' and the latter 'statistical or hospital', we can see advantages and disadvantages in each. When there is but one instructor, usually unsupported by the large and complicated apparatus of a hospital organisation, the latest discoveries in physiology and pathology are apt to suffer some neglect; there is pressure exerted on both teacher and pupil by the environment of the home to consider before all things the present emergency, including the social and financial strain of having a sick member on their hands. The patient is seen in the world in which he lives. Under such conditions it is admittedly not easy to examine in detail the workings of his various organs, but it is difficult not to see the way his life is tied in bonds of affection and dislike, in aspiration and despair, to his relatives and the social group of which he is a member. The apprentice to the general practitioner penetrated into the home and stood both to gain and to lose by that medical relationship.

A patient sent to hospital (to use the usual phrase) enters an unfamiliar region of social space. Within that organised system of research and therapy the easiest objects of study are the 'parts of the machine'—

those portions of the individual patient which are most susceptible to test and measurable reaction. In such an environment of isolation from the personal and social forces which act upon the personality it is difficult to get a comprehensive understanding of the personality of the patient. An over-all view is a greater achievement of clinical synthesis in a hospital than in a house; a thoroughgoing mechanistic analysis of the patient is more difficult in the home than in the ward.

The task of medical education is to develop fully the capacity both for clinical synthesis and for mechanistic analysis.[1]

(5) Post-war period

Subsequent experience has reinforced the change of emphasis and increased awareness of the social pressures. The growing study of stress led to the rapid accumulation of evidence that the normal function of a part or a bodily system may alter in response to stress, and that irreversible damage may occur.[2] Environmental concepts and the social life of the patient became of growing importance in medicine and surgery. The *British Medical Journal* commented in a leader:

Even if psychosomatic factors merely aggravate, rather than initiate, organic disease, nevertheless the psychosomatic school of medicine has made a useful contribution to contemporary thought. Psychosomatic medicine essentially is not a speciality, but a point of view, and an approach which applies equally to medical and surgical problems. It is basic medicine, which has needed re-emphasis.[3]

We live, too, within a contracting world. We meet Muslims and Jews, Hindus and Chinese; Africans come to Britian and the British travel abroad. Before our own eyes we see that people live by different rules, have different customs and ideals.

Technical aid from industrialised countries has been, time and again, frustrated in achieving its object by differences in the way of life between donors and recipients. Experts meet internationally with a quite unprecedented frequency, and discover not only a

[1] *B.M.J.* 2 (1947), 363.
[2] See H. Selye in *J. Clin. Endocrin.* 6 (1946), 117, and 'The Physiology and Pathology of Exposure to Stress', *Acta Endocrinologica* (Montreal, 1950); H. G. Woolff, *Stress and Disease* (Springfield, Ill., 1953).
[3] *B.M.J.* 2 (1951), 1137.

community of interest but also divisions in matters of ideals. In the West, they return home to countries where something of the order of half of the general practitioner's work is attributed to some form of mental malaise. Because of the cross-cultural influences to which the experts have been exposed, they necessarily come to question the social context within which they had hitherto seen their own speciality at home. They lift their eyes to the wider horizon and are reminded that the whole post-war world, Communist and non-Communist, is involved in a conflict of ideology. By 1951 L. W. Simmons could say in New York:

> Now, as we have said, there is mounting conviction on the part of medical leadership that knowledge of the socio-cultural dynamics of disease is often essential to diagnosis and prognosis, and all but indispensable to a preventive or therapeutic program...an increasing number of illnesses all along the way from pediatrics to geriatrics are now legitimate suspects for psycho-social and culturally derived complications; and that in the interests of good medical care these factors can no longer be ignored or neglected. The present scientific concern for this problem is such that a very warm and friendly attitude on the part of the attending physician, and an artful bedside manner, is no longer regarded as an adequate substitute for systematic knowledge with respect to these forces.[1]

At that same conference on Research in Public Health, W. T. Vaughan issued an important warning:

> From our experience at the Harvard School of Public Health in trying to pursue family research in a community mental health program, we have found it extremely difficult to use successfully the existing tools which the social sciences have to offer. I think that we are now at least seeing what the trouble is. When we originally went into the social scientists' storehouse of tools, we went in with the notion that they would be able to provide us with the necessary conceptual schemes and tools to apply to the problems in which we were interested. Actually, I think we have found that it does not work that way. Social scientists later, after we have worked for a year or two together, say, 'You have to tell us what it is you want to know and *together* we have to develop new concepts and tools to fit that particular problem.'

[1] 'A Frame of Reference for Family Research in Problems of Medical Care', in *Research in Public Health* (Milbank Memorial Fund, New York, 1952), pp. 172–3.

It seems to me throughout the discussion..., the help of the social sciences was stressed as being needed, but as yet we have not really come to grips here in this room as to how that help is going to come, and how to really integrate the important variables studied by social scientists into our family research program.[1]

There is increased social awareness, if not necessarily increased social skill.

Scientific thought and social pressures

Even the ivory tower is dependent upon its environment, and the common practices of a people find their way into scientific thought. Let us look at someone taking a pulse. He is using an ancient method of investigation; he counts over but a short period of time. If his count is to have meaning, it must be referred to some norm; he is using, as thousands of others do in different walks of life, a notion basic to what after centuries of use became the theory of sampling. Again, consider the traditional cures of taking plants, roots, seeds, concoctions for controlling the behaviour of the human body; from these habits there have developed the refinements of the chemist and biochemist. The real achievement was to make explicit something that had for long been implicit.

Imagine that by some technique the human ability which has been at work in a great teaching hospital throughout its history could be extracted, and put into another kind of culture; a Brahmin one, where there can be no experimenting with the dead, for they must be burnt quickly. It may well be that the ability which expressed itself in pharmacy could be put to work in a very similar if not identical way; but clearly there would be difficulties with the ability which in western culture expressed itself in and around the anatomy school. In a culture where the knife is prohibited, much of the ability might never express itself at all. Some of it, however, might express itself in other ways: the topographical knowledge of the human body might greatly increase, or perhaps men might earlier have concentrated upon the possibility of exploring the body with light, and thus might earlier have developed X-rays.

[1] In *Research in Public Health*, pp. 223–4.

We live and move and think as creatures within our own culture. In Lisbon, mechanical contraception does not enter the Portuguese doctor's head when he is considering his advice, not because he is incompetent, but merely because, like us all, he lives within his own way of life.

At the end of the war, Allied scientists refused to look at the information collected from certain freezing experiments performed in the concentration camps. Their refusal was not on the ground that the experimenters were incompetent, nor that they had cheated, but because for the Allied scientists there were overriding forces of morals and ethics which made such experiments disgusting. As civilised people, perhaps they would have said—as products of their own culture—they knew better.

The experiments had, however, been performed. The men who performed them were trained in scientific methods. What is the difference between these two bodies of men? Do they differ *qua* scientists; or is it not the fact that whereas for the Allied scientists there were cultural pressures prohibiting those actions, for the German scientists those pressures were either not there, or were inhibited by equal and opposite forces? The German and Allied scientists, the Portuguese and Nonconformist doctors, the Brahmin herbalists and Scottish surgeons, are creatures of their environment.

PROFESSIONAL FRAME OF REFERENCE

Nevertheless, if the Portuguese doctor is Portuguese in his way of life, he differs markedly from the rest of the Portuguese in consequence of his medical training, and his thinking has marked similarities, professionally at least, to that of his Nonconformist medical acquaintance in Birmingham. Within the general framework of his traditional thought and feeling the professional person builds up a highly specialised frame of reference; and because he does so, he comes to be socially useful.

The importance of different environments in moulding attitudes and general outlook is obvious to any student. On his arrival at college the structure and composition of this new world seems to him quite new, standards of value and achievement differ widely from those of his immediate past, and his own position is entirely altered. William James remarked that a baby's consciousness must be a booming buzzing confusion; so too can a hospital be on the first day one enters its doors. It is not easy at the end of one's career to recapture that confusion—our thinking and feeling is governed by the complicated map, plan or frame of reference which we have built up.

Much the same is true of the doctor's professional knowledge. There was a time for every student when he first put on professional spectacles, when he first attempted to look at a person like a doctor looking at a patient. The truth was that on this first occasion people did not look any different, and the student drew the sensible conclusion that he had yet to acquire his professional knowledge. At the end of his career, however, when he looks through his professional spectacles, people *do* look different; he sees at least some of the things which he is taught to see.

This specialised knowledge which is to be socially useful creates its own difficulties in understanding people. It is hard to recapture our own buzzing confusion of early days, hard to see illness except through professional spectacles—without our own frame of reference. The late Sir James Spence said that in the art of consultation, before explanation and advice could be given to a patient (or parent), three diagnoses must be made—namely of the disease, of the concept of the disease in the mind of the patient, and of the patient's capacity to understand the explanation and follow the advice.[1]

The doctor is useful to the mother because he has been trained to think about her child in a way different from hers. His way of thinking, however, his facility in thinking, and his familiarity with disease, may well create a barrier between himself and his understanding of the mother's problem.

O. G. Simmons recounts how the redeployment of nurses in Chile from the ante-natal and well-baby clinics to home-visiting led to a virtual breakdown of communication between doctor and

[1] Sir J. C. Spence, *B.M.J.* I (1949), 629.

patient in the clinics. When the doctor asked the patient if she understood the instruction, she invariably gave a perfunctory affirmative reply:

Most Chilean doctors are of upper-class background, whereas those served by the health centers ordinarily belong to the lower classes. Patients defer to the authority of the doctor as an upper-class person as much as to his authority as a medical expert....Nurses, on the other hand, generally come from the Chilean lower or middle classes and are accorded less prestige but more confidence....Many doctors believe the capacity of people to understand and thus to co-operate is directly related to their formal education and economic status. One doctor said...he measured the mental capacity of his patients by the number of years of schooling they had and equated illiteracy with mental deficiency.[1]

Many men, while able to accept the aphorism that the British and Americans are divided by a common language, are reluctant to accept—and sometimes altogether fail to understand—that the very skill of a lawyer or doctor or priest can build a barrier against an understanding of other people.

Yet it is readily recognised that speech provides a course for some of the most powerful of environmental forces. Now the sciences necessarily create their own language with its own over-tones, links and discipline of thought: there is accepted, with its vocabulary, the rational and causal approach. The acceptance of this approach is insisted upon from early life, to become 'second nature' in the rational scientist; but such an approach does not hold, for example, in tribal Africa. Demonstrate that the mosquito carries malaria and the traditional African response will be, 'But why did that mosquito bite me?' The scientist thinks the question irrelevant; the tribal African thinks the scientist abandons his approach at the point where it becomes interesting and intensely relevant.

Thought can be disciplined in other than scientific ways: lawyers, poets, rabbis, musicians, may not split a single atom; but who is to deny that they have created their own languages, with overtones,

[1] 'The Clinical Team in a Chilean Health Center' in B. D. Paul (ed.), *Health, Culture and Community* (New York, 1955), p. 339.

2-2

links and discipline of thought? Each one of these professional people, like the tribal African, leads his own life provided by his environment. His thoughts and feelings, ideas and ideals may not be those of the scientists. A considerable effort may be demanded of the scientist to conceive of life in other people's terms. The effort must be made, however, if the scientist is to understand how the behaviour of people with different outlook, with different environmental experience, coheres.

In general practice a man is his own interpreter, his own investigator. E. M. Creak wrote concerning the nervous child:

...the doctor needs time to gain his facts. It will repay him to study feelings and family attitudes rather than actions and he may well find that the patient's or the parent's own words will tell him more than his own questions. His conclusions will be strengthened by his intimate knowledge of the background in which his child patient lives.

And again,

Indeed, the art of history-taking lies not so much in leaving no stone unturned as in creating an informal situation in which a troubled parent will feel free enough to admit to herself, and to the doctor, something of what is worrying her...and a good diagnosis depends neither on flair nor on training so much as on good relationships and a good history.[1]

[1] *B.M.J.* 2 (1951), 287.

CHAPTER II

PHYSICIAN AND
NEIGHBOURHOOD

The doctor in practice cannot take the anthropologist's care to
select the area which is to be the subject of his investigation. It is
found for him: the object must be to understand the way of life of
the children who are already in his waiting-room. R. J. F. H.
Pinsent has written:

> The family doctor cannot live the lives and experience the emotions
> of all the families and persons for whose health he is responsible, but he
> can and must find out all he can about their way of life, at work and at
> home, and all that this entails....It is background knowledge such as
> this that gives balance to the work of the doctor in general practice and
> differentiates his work from that of the consultant, to whom it is denied
> by virtue of his isolation in hospital. Only the general practitioner is
> able to add up the domestic, physical and economic stresses that may at
> the same time affect an individual or a family.[1]

There is no commonly accepted way of examining a neighbourhood. No proposal is made here for a method of routine examination. The aim is, however, proceeding from the considerations
of the previous chapter, to encourage the doctor, aware of the need
to have some understanding of social life, to enter the field reasonably confident that he can make some appraisal.

FRAME OF REFERENCE

It is necessary for the doctor to examine his own approach to the
neighbourhood, to study and make as explicit as possible the frame
of reference which is to be used. Some fact may well be already
known and the refinement and extension of it will pre-determine
part of the frame of reference. There will also be much opinion, not

[1] *An Approach to General Practice* (London, 1953), p. 87.

necessarily well ordered, but constituting his expectations—the product of information or hearsay and of his own temperament, habits, morals and beliefs. This product is the most important part of the frame of reference and the most difficult to describe. There is real advantage in attempting to make it as explicit as possible.

Secondly, records are usually available and should be consulted. In Britain it is comparatively easy to obtain information of a geographical—structural and climatic—nature. Easy too, to find guide-book information, giving some historical picture, together with sociological data of economic and industrial development and land use. These, together with photographs, maps, the statistical information on the constitution of the population, its age, class, sex and marital status, distribution, densities, etc., coupled with the information contained within the reports of the medical officer of health, give facts to be erected into a more or less coherent whole upon the vague basis of attitudes, stereotypes and expectations.

Application

Upon entering the new neighbourhood, there take place swiftly many mental processes which are not easily recalled. Time is spent identifying the things that are already known, and much time is spent too in comparisons: 'Bigger than I thought, older than I thought'; and also in recognising aspects of local life not yet expected (and very easily and quickly forgotten after adaptation is made): 'It's noisier/quieter, more smelly/fresh, the people are smaller/taller, better/worse-dressed, uglier/more handsome than I thought.'

If the way of life differs markedly from that to which the doctor was formerly accustomed, some of his own assumptions, parts of his own frame of reference which before were not explicit readily appear. After a few days in a remote rural area, it may occur to a man that he has not wound up his watch: that his assumptions about punctuality and his notions of time are inappropriate there.

In proportion as a new community resembles his own, he will find it increasingly hard to appreciate and allow for differences in outlook, or to recognise the basis from which his own outlook is derived. The doctor's notions about clock time, for example, may lead to anger and misunderstanding in a poor working-class area of an industrial British town, or in cities overseas where watches are often a personal decoration rather than a governing instrument.

After a while he will find it possible to identify dwellings and to describe their immediate surroundings; to recognise other buildings and to describe how what is done there indicates the life of the neighbourhood; to describe, in general terms, how a living is earned, how leisure is spent, how the neighbourhood acts corporately, for its own comfort and convenience, to meet disaster, to forestall it, and to rejoice.

He will then see the dwellings, in their variety, within this context, and upon entering them will recognise some at least of the equipment and understand the general disposition of goods, so that he can give an account of how the physical dwelling is converted into a household. Observation will show something of the daily rhythm of events, and that will reveal longer cycles of weeks and seasons and years both in the household and generally in the neighbourhood. Within this general pattern, the individual goes through his own life-cycle.

Infants and children there will move through the life-cycle with its own internal rhythm within the environment, and, in Britain, within a swiftly moving culture. All these things, of which but the merest hint has been given here, will come to bear upon them. He will, however, still be a long way from understanding whole orders of forces that come to bear upon them. He will not be much further advanced than to be able to speculate upon what he expects to be the differences between growing up within this new environment and growing up in the one he knows best.

Comparison

The importance of what may conveniently be called the physical environment—the climatic, geographical and ecological facts—and man's response to them by way of shelter, clothing and food is understood, and great progress has been made to control the physical environment within the British Isles. As fewer problems are presented to the doctor that arise from ignorance of this physical environment, relatively more, and especially in the persons of children, are presented to him which arise directly from the way of life. To understand these problems we must appreciate as best we can that way of life. The doctor, if he is to understand what is presented to him, is increasingly compelled to attempt to identify the most difficult group of factors within that context: neither bricks nor micro-organisms, but morals and beliefs, axioms and assumptions.

It is difficult to bridge the gap between describing a way of life and understanding the experience of living that way of life; but a bridge can be created. First, in the process of observation and description, the doctor's original assumptions about the way of life have almost certainly been modified, and these changes should be identified. Secondly, an attempt may be made to assess how child-life in the new environment differs from that of the doctor's own environment. Some general comparison can be made between, say, what appear to be the differences in the general standard of ante-natal care in the two environments, in maternal diet, in the kind and amount of supervision which the mother receives, in physical activities and, perhaps, in attitudes to the need for rest. The comparison should then proceed from the birth to the establishment of the infant, to his childhood and school days. The comparisons should include at each stage an assessment of differences in equipment and routine, differences in the hazards (physical, economic and mental), differences in relationships with other members of the family, both child and adult, and with people outside the family. Carefully done and in some detail, the two environments can be seen by the doctor each in the light of the other.

New insights

This permits the third and important step. The practitioner may accept himself as a creature of his own environment, experienced in its way of living, and now faced with questions concerning the experience of life in the new environment that are entirely his own. These questions are the product of the interplay of his own environmental experience and his observation of a different way of life. The questions, by their origin, are comparative ones. By working through the mental exercise of transposing a household from his own environment with all its belongings to the new, questions can be multiplied, and at the same time new insights gained. Starting with the material equipment and its disposition, he will quickly realise the importance of relating human behaviour to its social context. The possibility arises, for example, that husbands and wives, mothers and fathers, have functions which vary with the rules, prohibitions, demands and expectations which are made. Within the general culture the life of the neighbourhood has its place: within the neighbourhood the family finds its place and function. The daily round contributes to the larger rhythm, the individual progresses from birth to death. The individuals, unique in their creation, experience inevitably and individually the pressures of their environment, producing their expectations from life, producing what they ask of life and what life asks of them. The practitioner comes to learn, in effect, that though the words father, mother, husband, wife, son, daughter, sister, brother, may have precise biological meaning, they tell us little of the individual's experience of life, what society demands of him, what he, in turn, expects of society, and how his individual and unique endowment comes to be related with what is after all his unique environment.

We see the individual in a new perspective and in consequence can see anew whole areas of knowledge. We see something of the difficulty of applying the conclusions of the textbook to the practical everyday world. In particular two problems of application are illuminated. The first is that however logical, inevitable and impersonal the effects, say, of war or disease may appear to be to the uninvolved observer, the historian or public health officer, the reactions and adaptations of people who experience these events are determined by their way of life. The second, apart from catastrophe, is that what people feel to be their needs do not necessarily appear to the observer to be either desirable or necessary consequences of the facts as he understands them.

Social problems concern people. One can say that a town lacks drains, that cholera there is a public health problem: but it is sick men, women and children who present themselves at the surgery. Their illness can only be explained by the physician within its social context in environmental terms; but pain and anxiety are what count for the patients.

The problems that catch the attention of the uninvolved observer may not be the felt, recognised problems of the society. It might strike an observer, for example, that daily deaths and injuries from road accidents exceed those from war and disease, and he might well wonder why it is that people devote so much energy to the avoidance of casualties in war, so much energy to the conquest of disease, so little energy to the control of a regularly recurring hazard. As he became closer acquainted with people's ways and ideals, and with their high regard for children, he might well be amazed to discover that to children the home is even more dangerous than the road. He would be right to conclude that this society has no strongly felt need to tackle the problem. He might be moved to persuade the people; but changing the ways of an individual or a society is no easy thing. Tobacco smoking increases in spite of increased price and the cancer scare. He might note, too, that water is chlorinated for children to swim in, but that they breathe impure air for many hours a day in the classroom. Although the consequences are known, and some control possible, it almost seems that care is taken to ensure that the children are collected there in the winter months and dispersed in the summer months. If he were moved to do something about this, he would soon find that there is no felt problem, that there would be resistance to change. The argument would be put forward that the changes involved are enormous and expensive. That is to say, society is prepared to pay the price—not a consciously calculated one, but one that arises from the nature of events, and thus is there to be paid. Societies may endure scourges because they do not know what else to do. Scurvy, avitaminosis, and death from starvation were the common concomitants of a hard winter in this country until within the living memory of a very old man. These were but a part of life, and became problems to be attacked when the weapon came to hand in our own day, so that, for example, only ten cases of scurvy have been seen at Great Ormond Street in five years.[1]

Secondly, rational procedures are not always acceptable to a people. Even in our own society we do not always see the causal connection in disease: 'It is chastening to note that evidence of the epidemic relations of a defect which had until so recently been regarded as accidental was available in census reports and institutional data for anyone who cared to look for it during the last 50 years.'[2]—This concerning rubella and congenital deafness. Rational procedures based upon this discovered connection offend no one. The rationale of any or all of the methods of mechanical contraception may be irrefutable; but the Catholic does not, therefore, abandon his beliefs and adopt these methods. However logical the procedures of vaccination and analgesia in child-birth may be, they were not guaranteed thereby an immediate, unhesitating acceptance within the British Isles.

Again, and further afield: a health-team visited a remote tribe in Southern Africa.[3] It was seen at once that the people were infected with tuberculosis. Now, it would seem the simplest thing to the outsider to say so and to add that the disease is controllable, and then, surely, everybody falls in happily and in due course out goes tuberculosis. Events did not work out thus. The Zulus knew they were infected, they had notions of infection, they knew the infection was spread by persons. But they were convinced that the evil infection was consciously spread by evil people. They knew it to be work of witches. Their problem was witches, and witches they sought. To explain that the loving mother was infecting her infant presented the physician with a nice problem. He might—and with reason in the context—find himself labelled an evil, malicious trouble-maker, if not hounded out as a witch himself. The social problem was evil persons. The problem may from the point of view

---

[1] G. Howells, P. E. S. Palmer & W. H. St J. Brooks, *B.M.J.* 2 (1954), 1143.
[2] *B.M.J.* 2 (1951), 1511.
[3] J. Cassel, 'A Comprehensive Health Program among South African Zulus', in B. D. Paul (ed.), *Health, Culture and Community*.

of the uninvolved outsider be misconceived, in the sense that his mechanical logical remedy is excluded by the local formulation and the feeling people invest therein.

Assisting individuals within their culture needs an understanding of, and feeling for, their way of life. The very practical matter of treating a sick or troubled child calls for a firm grasp of theoretical principles not the least of which is that man and child, physician and patient, are like all life, interactive with and interdependent upon their several environments.

CHAPTER III

NEIGHBOURHOOD AND CHILD

Observing a family, watching it at work, we may ask three inter-related questions. How are the primary needs of man met? What culture and traditions are consciously observed and taught? What, in performing these two, and otherwise, is passively learnt?

Man and his child need shelter, clothing and food. It is not my intention here to pursue the matters of housing and food, which are more appropriately subjects of public health and nutrition.

It is useful to distinguish between the objective and subjective components of a way of life. We have begun with the objective components: brick, mortar, and equipment; and also behaviour, the way people earn their living, and the way husbands, wives, mothers and fathers behave. These may be used to understand the subjective components: what goes on in people's heads, hearts, and minds.

We shall consider the folkways, mores, laws and ethical principles, how they come to bear upon a family and how they are brought to bear upon the infant in the home. In the following chapter the child's experience of these forces outside the home and at school are considered, and subsequently the methods of enforcement are dealt with.

Folkways may be described, perhaps, as custom—saying 'please' and 'thank you', using a handkerchief, a knife and fork, eating foods in a certain order. Their violation by adults will bring, not so much punishment, but expressions of surprise, contempt or disgust from others. Children acquire them in part passively, in part by explicit teaching.

Mores have a stronger emotional investment, and their violation by an adult will provoke protest and sometimes action. The un-married mother, for example, suffers from breaking them. There is no sharp division between folkways and mores; but failure on the part of their children to observe the mores will tend to create greater anxiety in parents than a breach of the folkways. It may indicate either that the parents are unable to care for and protect the child or that the child is in some way abnormal.

Laws are rules which have some formal recognition and procedure, generally with specified agents for their enforcement, either by way of public control, or by punishment for their breach, or both. There is a general tendency for mores to be formulated into laws. But ethical principles are characteristically regarded as non-human in origin. They may come from God or gods, from Nature or Reason. They establish what is good and evil, right and wrong. Their actual exposition is relatively unimportant, for every member of a society has early embedded within him the value-system of his people. A breach is ordinarily a sin, and according to the gravity with which it is regarded, it may require penance or expiation or it may be irremediable, in which case damnation follows.

Folkways, mores, laws and ethics are all interwoven, and sometimes in conflict. Together they make demands upon individuals and groups; with the demands are associated the individual's expectations, and founded on these there arise the assumptions and beliefs of the individual. Here these matters are considered in the restricted context of rearing children.

The economic conditions of the home can be ascertained without much difficulty. But what is far more important is the cultural outlook of the parents, the daily influence that they and their acquaintances will exercise on the child's developing incentives, and the emotional tension that may be set up in the mind of the child when the atmosphere of the home is unfavourable to intellectual work or to stable development of character—in short, the whole sociological background of the individual child....

I would therefore urge that far more attention be paid to what is somewhat vaguely termed 'social psychology'—especially the study of class differences and of social attitudes and their differential influence on the younger generation...a psychologist...who lives for a time in a settlement in the slums or as a guest in the house of a Limehouse dock-labourer or Bermondsey coster-monger (as every intending educational psychologist should do), will find the customs and ideals almost as strange as if he was on an anthropological expedition to the Torres Straits; and he will be surprised to learn how his own behaviour and vocabulary strikes his candid proletarian friends as full of fossilized symptoms of a 'bourgeois mentality', which he himself supposed he has sloughed off long ago.[1]

LOCAL NORMS

The first task, then, is to establish the local norms of family relationships, habits, morals, and so on, and to distinguish them from those of one's own home and upbringing. The variation in local norms may be due to many factors. Occupation accounts for some.

Fishing and seafaring folk are bound to have a different way of life from, say, farming and mining communities; shop-keeping provides different conditions from office-work, shift-work from seasonal trades, long distance transport from the making of daily rounds—and with the occupation there will go different family relationships, habits and possibly morals. Families are made up of unique individuals: the individual is unique because of his genetic and environmental individuality.

The Rev. Gilbert Dawson is now in his early fifties and since the war has been the devoted vicar of Barron, a prosperous residential town on the south coast. The living is a good one, the vicarage, built in 1939, is substantial but efficient and comfortable. The vicar is married; there are two sons, aged 16 years and 14 years.

He has a good deal to do—not that he complains; but there is a regular weekly round, which keeps him tied to his parish. He had not had a holiday for some years—summers are busy because he lives on the coast and in the poorer weather he is disinclined to go away, mainly because the parish activities of the darker evenings need him and interest him.

After long persuasion, he took a few days off to fish.

He had slept at home every night for nearly four years; for years he had been daily at home and in the parish.

It was a new sensation for the two boys to wake up and find their father was not about the place. The older one decided the gap might well be filled. In the course of the day he said to some friends, 'My Dad has gone away for a few days fishing. We are giving a party. Would you care to come?'

[1] Sir C. Burt, *Brit. J. Educ. Psychol.* XVII (1947), 2, 65.

It was a new sensation for the wife to wake up and find that her husband was not about. They had shared the same double bed every night since he was demobbed. She stretched herself and found herself saying, 'What a lot of room there is in a double bed when you are alone.'

Compare this with an occurrence in the family next door.

Frank Harrington had bought the house next to the vicarage at the end of the war. The houses were identical. He, too, was married and had two sons of a similar age to those of the vicar. He had bought the house with an eye to retirement, for he was the captain of a liner.

On the day Frank Harrington was due home from a long cruise, his sixteen-year-old said to his friends, 'My Dad is coming home tonight and we are giving a party.' His wife woke up to say, 'Frank is coming home to me tonight.'

In these two families, from the mere fact of the men's jobs, there must be different habits and relationships between husbands and wives, between mothers and sons. The mother in the sailor's family must take decisions, for example, which in the other family are within the father's province.

It is necessary to know something of environmental circumstances if one is to understand the problem of the individual. Rowntree and Lavers point out that in the Rhondda Valley great emphasis is still placed on sexual morality.[1] The fact that Gwyneth in the valley is pregnant clearly presents Gwyneth and everyone who wants to help her with a very different problem from that of Sylvia who is pregnant and unmarried. Sylvia is from Jamaica and she has been living with her chap, also from Jamaica, for about a year, in Brixton. We know nothing about Gwyneth or Sylvia as persons. When we come to know them as unique individuals we shall understand their personal problems only if these individuals are seen within their social context.

DEMANDS

All societies make demands upon their individuals. There are rules to be obeyed, duties performed, conventions to be observed, the way of life, within prescribed limits, to be followed. Those demands

[1] B. S. Rowntree and G. R. Lavers, *English Life and Leisure* (London, 1951), p. 204.

within the British Isles, which themselves sustain a complicated, illogical, old, and changing system of social struture and economic life, vary markedly from place to place, and ultimately from family to family.

Local folkways present themselves: 'It's done' to contribute to wreaths, give Christmas presents, tip, stand rounds of drinks; and then on to the things which are necessary for 'keeping up with the Joneses', whether it be in terms of car, pram, television set, holidays, fur coat, children, dancing classes, window ornaments, whitening of steps or washing the area of pavement immediately before the threshold. Respectability and keeping up with the Joneses, if not the only integrating forces, help local norms to cohere.

Demands of folkways and mores upon mothers vary from place to place.

Jane was London-born and married a Canadian when he was working as a ship's steward. He left the sea and settled down to farming in Canada some eighty miles from the nearest town. When visited Jane had one child, a girl about a year old. She complained that for the past week the child 'had spots—red and angry ones'. She had put cold cream on them, but they had spread, her child was restive and she had resolved to 'call' the doctor (i.e. telephone him). The doctor was in the town eighty miles away. He was prepared to accept the mother's description of her daughter; and, further, prepared to instruct her as to the treatment for the condition.

Now tell this same simple story about Jane's twin sister Jean, who married a sheet-metal worker and lived in East London. Her child had spots and Jean treated them with cold cream for a week. The spots spread, her child was restive and she had resolved to take her to the doctor. The moment the doctor examined the child, he rose and said with marked disapproval, 'Why didn't you bring her before?' The social organisation in the two places differs markedly. If Jean was the sort of girl whom the doctor in London would regard as an intelligent and co-operative mother, and she had married the Canadian, she might well have been a failure in a remote Canadian homestead—she might ask the doctor to motor a round trip of 160 miles to come to look at a napkin rash.

The city mother is at the receiving end of specialisation. There is a demand made upon her, not that she should approach her children with confidence, but that she should come to know that some say it matters when you pot your children and how, whether they suck their thumbs, or wet the bed; that some say ordinary children should not be taught to read until they are six, that fairy stories are bad; that there is a whole array of doctors, psychologists, educationists, all devoted to children. There is a demand made upon her not that mother should know best, that she should be a confident mother; but that she should know her way about the specialities and how to bring them to bear—and early—upon her child.

There is no oddity about parents loving their children. Where, exceptionally, love is not found, one looks for an individual cause. How that love is expressed is determined by the rules of the society. Some loving parents send their little boys of eight away to school for some forty weeks of the year.

Parents loved their children two generations ago. Literate, and with a copy of *Enquire Within*, Jean's grandparents had confidence to deal with problems of making a will, landlord and tenant, master and servant, the wife's change of life and all those things about their children which they felt could not be solved by the light of nature. Their other granddaughter Jane, in Canada, takes the *Parents' Magazine* and possesses Dr Spock's excellent book.[1] Jean lives differently from either Jane or their grandparents. 'There has never been an age' said the *Report of the Committee on Maladjusted Children,*

in which more was known about children, but it is also true that there has never been an age in which parents had less confidence in their own powers to handle their children. In time past parents relied on instinct and common sense; but in the complexity of modern civilization these are overlaid or mistrusted, and popular books on psychology are no substitute. Some of the common beliefs about the behaviour and development of children are very misleading, and many parents become anxious if their children do not develop with the speed and behave in the manner expected.[2]

[1] B. Spock, *Baby and Child Care* (London, 1955).
[2] H.M.S.O. (1955), p. 132.

Demands are made upon all the members of the family. Wars and periods of swift cultural change bring about alterations in these demands, and some individuals are more adaptable than others, but clearly differences between husband and wife, between the married couple and their neighbourhood, of class, religion, race or up-bringing, contribute to difficulties in responding to local demands. Sometimes changes which are eagerly sought bring their own com-plications. Reared in an overcrowded dwelling in inner London, and having started their married life there, the couple move off (at last) to a new housing estate. New demands are made, inevitably, on husband and wife. Not all can respond adequately; not all find the imagined happiness; not all stay.[1] Some of the effects of swift cultural change upon families may be illustrated by the Polish-speaking couple who came to settle in a country district here. To them is born a son, a bright boy, who, now aged thirteen, is going by bus to the local grammar school. English-speaking from birth, a British subject by birth, he knows more of the British way of life than his parents ever can. How, in that family, can there be an assumption of the wisdom of the old, that mother knows best? How is parental discipline maintained; how does the family cohere? Or compare:

(i) John, aged four, is the son of a chartered accountant. His mother died when he was born. The home was kept going by the father's widowed mother, who was glad to make a home for her son and grandson, for she is still active and, until her husband—a successful barrister—had died two years previously, she had run a large house. Father is away on business a good deal. Grandmother is in sole charge, is fond of her grandson and he is doing very well.

(ii) Alan, nearly four, is the first-born of the Wilsons. Mrs Wilson, now twenty-five, the daughter of a successful barrister, had trained as a nursery-school teacher and married an accountant. She is fond of her son and he is doing very well.

Because of the difference in age of the two women, living within a swiftly moving culture, the environment differs markedly. What is right or wrong, nice, proper or good form, is by no means common to the two homes.

[1] See M. Young and P. Willmott, *Family and Kinship in East London* (London, 1957).

EXPECTATIONS

Closely related to what is demanded of one is what one expects. People are ordinarily not good witnesses about their expectations. A girl who is to marry tomorrow may say she expects from marriage a husband, love, a home, children. She will dismiss the inquirer as unnecessarily realistic if he attempts to break down these replies by questions about washing up, making beds, cleaning shoes, mending, the number of knives and forks, the amount of money for the household budget now, and two, three and four decades hence. A glance, however, at the home she has prepared shows that she has given detailed thought to some of these things, and the answers to some of the others are implied by the dwelling itself and its equipment. A year or so hence she may well be saying, 'he wants a servant/mother/nanny, not a wife. He takes no notice of me/he won't leave me alone. It hasn't worked out. You don't expect your husband to....'

W. G. Fox and F. D. O. Collins recount some interesting differences in expectations in marriage between older (45–60) women attending women's afternoon groups in the older working-class areas of Hull, and younger (20–35) women from the newer housing estates.[1] They found that generalisations put forward and strongly supported in one or a number of groups are either not introduced or dismissed as invalid by other groups. The investigators remarked that older women frequently spoke with apparent disregard for possible loss of prestige of the indignities and humiliations (frequently involving physical ill-treatment) suffered during the early years of marriage, and their statements were invariably accepted by the rest of the groups as typical. They saw the woman as completely dependent on the man, and their roles at home quite separate. The older groups were virtually united in their scorn for the modern husband of the more 'democratic' marriage, and among the younger ones there were frequent expressions of envy at the more clearly differentiated domestic pattern of the past. The investigators judged today's marital aims to be more diffused and personalised,

[1] In *Social Service Quarterly* (winter, 1956), p. 116.

the first requirement being 'happiness', and they see a more ready acceptance of divorce as a way out of an unhappy (as opposed to an intolerable) marital situation, the individual having the right to end it because he is unhappy and to seek happiness elsewhere.

The hostility of the older group was directed particularly against the young married couple without children, and their prevailing attitude was one of grave foreboding as to the ultimate result of the constant easing of material conditions. The younger women said, 'What do our parents know about marriage today? They are always on about money coming in but they don't talk so much about the amount we have to pay out.' There was a good deal of evidence that the modern parent was aware of the non-material needs of children, but the child was not merely important in his own right but almost equally important as a visible indication of the quality of the relationship between his parents, taking his place along with the television set and the washing-machine as outward evidence of its success.

ASSUMPTIONS AND BELIEFS

With some knowledge of the structure of social life, it is possible for a study of language to expose axioms, self-evident assumptions and beliefs that are current.

Saida's father, a Pakistani, was in the diplomatic service. He had brought his family from Karachi to London, and after a month or two to settle down, Saida, aged $3\frac{1}{2}$ years, had been sent to a nursery school. After her first term, father was asked what he made of his daughter now that she had been thus exposed to English influence. 'Oh she's all right,' he said, 'except she will say "thank you" to her mother and me.'

Mother and father do not expect to be thanked. Because the child is their daughter, it is axiomatic that they will give. The bond is emphasised by not thanking parents, but remembering to thank servants and more remote members of the family. Nevertheless, in Britain, the northern European custom of all the family, including father, thanking the mother before rising at the end of a meal, does not prevail—nor do the assumptions behind it.

Juan, aged 5 years, was at home in Madrid and had drawn a bed. Jaime, aged four and his brother, took the view that the pot under the bed was not an integral part of the drawing, said so, and suggested it be removed. 'No Señor', said Juan with finality.

Little boys who address each other as 'Señor' assume a personal dignity which the British adult who is addressed by his children as 'Tom' may neither believe in, nor be capable of attaining. British fathers are no longer called 'sir' by their children. Some are invariably 'Dad', but children often show a nice awareness of relationships, when, for example, a daughter may proceed from the equalitarian (or superior) intimacy of 'Tom' to the subordinate and dependent 'Daddy', the everyday 'Dad', then to the telephone question, 'Do you want to speak to Mr Jones?' on to the final nicety of 'Tom Jones, Esq.' on an envelope.

Slim White, aged seventeen years, an only child and a Londoner, was talking of household arrangements. 'Our Mum', he said, 'always gets up first.'

There were three members of this household: mother, father and himself; yet he used the possessive plural when speaking of his mother. This is a common form of local speech; yet it would appear from the facts that he would be precluded from using it. Perhaps both men call her 'Mum': perhaps she mothers father as well as son.

Mrs Cricknell, now middle-aged, has gone to the doctor 'about her inside'. In the course of talking to him—a burly, iron-grey, active man—she said, 'You must let your husband have his rights, doctor.'

Her reference to sexual intercourse left her neatly out of it— uninvolved; something men go in for and nothing to do with her. She did not seem to be 'outgoing' to the sexual relationship. Compare what she had to say with:

Mrs Garrett, aged 23 years, the wife of a transport worker and the mother of two young children. She announced the reason for her visit to the doctor as follows: 'I haven't seen anything for seven weeks, Doctor. I think I've fallen again.'

Perhaps she is pregnant again—fallen, like Eve, or slipped up, come to grief, had an accident. She has been looking for seven weeks.

She again does not appear to be outgoing, wanting to be fruitful and to multiply.

Contrast these two women with the young wives of professional men: the girl who says, 'We are not starting on a family for another two years', or 'If Jim gets the job we will start a family straight away'. Can one imagine that that girl pops into her husband's bed to let her husband have his rights? It seems that two quite different sets of relationships, habits, and morals are being exposed, based probably on different axioms, self-evident assumptions and beliefs.

Mrs Western had taught at a progressive school and had married the biology master. They had a twelve-year-old daughter and a ten-year-old son. Mrs Western consulted her doctor because the boy had begun to wet the bed. 'We are always quite frank with our children, Doctor. We answer their questions frankly. We never lock the bathroom door. They are both quite used to seeing me or my husband in the bath.'

Now it is clear that Mrs Western wants to tell the doctor something. If pressed, she would probably say that she aimed to be (and by her own lights was successful in being) truthful, factual, frank and free, that she hid nothing from her children. On consideration, can that really be so? Would she really, for example, be able to take a communal, open-air, evening tub with family and guests in a Japanese village? If she enjoyed the warm steamy privacy with her family of the Finnish *sauna*, could she also accompany her twelve-year-old daughter to the double privy of northern European country districts? Is everything—everything—she does with her husband exposed to her children's view—or does it just happen that the children have not been there when the couple have been telling not quite drawing-room stories, worrying about the future, about the children, quarrelling, enjoying sexual horseplay or copulating?

She is herself subject to social pressures, and in rearing her children she inevitably brings her own axioms, self-evident assumptions and beliefs to bear upon her children—as inevitably as they speak their mother tongue. It is quite unlikely that she is 'entirely frank': she probably means that her children are submitted to fewer conscious rules and prohibitions than she experienced in her own childhood. If there are fewer rules and prohibitions for the children

39

to learn, there is almost certainly a greater amount of passive learning to be done. She has consulted the doctor, for example, not because her son passes water, but because he passes it in a place of which she disapproves. And she disapproves for a whole complex of reasons, beginning perhaps with convenience and habit, and reaching down to her own axioms, self-evident assumptions, and beliefs.

These foregoing matters are considered as parts of the social context of the child, as factors in the environment which make him the child and person that he is. The observable habits, relationships and morals, the norms of local life, create demands and expectations, and they in turn give rise to assumptions and beliefs. Within their framework the child is reared, in countless detailed ways, continuing the folkways, mores and ethics of father and son, mother and daughter and largely determining their attitude to the law.

SOCIAL PRESSURES OF THE HOME

We do not easily recognise that, quite apart from whether there is a deep psychological effect upon the child, cultural factors enter into his earliest handling. The advocates of breast-feeding are certainly aware that fashion among women can be either their enemy or ally; they know, too, that the possibility of employing a wet-nurse changes with the decades and, in Europe, may range from the next to impossible to the quite usual; that demand-feeding may or may not be a local norm. I shall not attempt a detailed description of the pressures brought to bear upon the infant in his home, but I shall single out a few for illustration.

Cleanliness

The notions of cleanliness practised in British homes are not abstractions of science; but, basically, common ways of behaving. Babies are bathed. British people bath. British children share baths. The Duke of Windsor in his autobiography assures us that he shared a tin bath in his childhood. A moment's thought of what is dislodged from the body and dissolved, mixed with the water, and then more or less evenly distributed throughout the water by body movement, gives point to the Muslim's objection to baths and preference for showers. It illuminates the order in which children are taught to apply the soap, and perhaps, on reflection, reveals our own established habit. Care is taken not to wash all of the orifices of a female child with the same vigour; that the Chinese domestic knows of British parental desires in the matter, and that the little girl herself learns these differences.

Both boys and girls must be taught 'not to handle themselves'. The teaching may be by explicit prohibition, or it may be acquired by passive learning. A difficulty arises with the uncircumcised boy. Hygiene teaches that the glans must be washed; but the boy is to acquire the habit of not handling it. The revelation of retraction among the otherwise well-cared-for uncircumcised discloses this conflict. So perhaps, too, does the tradition of circumcision. Some twenty-four per cent of all males are circumcised in the British Isles; but among the public school-university group, the percentage is probably as high as eighty per cent and among the working class as low as ten per cent. MacCarthy, Douglas and Mogford found in a national sample of four-year-old children that thirty-nine per cent of the sons of the professional classes and twenty-two per cent of the sons of manual workers were circumcised.[1]

It is with great reluctance that the British come to consider whether girls 'handle themselves'—whether they masturbate. Schoolgirl 'crushes' are readily and tolerantly recognised; but the possibility of physical contact is unrecognised in a way which would strike a purdah-girl as unrealistic.

Infants are taught to sit on the pot and then on the lavatory. This training is very different from that followed by Greek mothers, who train their children to defecate only when the baby is old enough to imitate the mother. 'And in other cultures learning to defecate is often a part of the process of identification with the mother: the child, when able to walk, goes with the mother when she goes to defecate, and acts as she acts.'[2] Toilet-training is not

---

[1] D. MacCarthy, J. W. B. Douglas and C. Mogford, *B.M.J.* 2 (1952), 755.
[2] M. Mead (ed.), *Cultural Patterns and Technical Change* (U.N.E.S.C.O. 1955), p. 215.

mentioned in the two current Greek manuals on child care.[1] In a country where watches are adornments and clocks furnishings, but where the pressure of 'modern' living is being felt in the towns, the manuals, contrary to tradition, teach scheduled feeds and bed-time, and insist that the child should not go at its own pace.[2] At the same time they subscribe to traditional ways by devoting 'much space to character-training; obedience is taught first, almost from birth; it is the parents' task to mould the character of the child, to be firm and unyielding. Mothers are urged not to be indulgent or over-protective.'[3] Again (and on the ground of cleanliness), our children are taught not to handle faeces—all faeces, that is to say, except horse-dung, which among other things may be tested by hand for its nuttiness by the keen gardener. The flushing of the lavatory is taught (where there is an abundance of water). The washing of hands is desirable (but no more extensive cleansing), although it appears from the efforts necessary to train adults who handle food, not taught. Boys learn to pass their water publicly, girls learn to do it privately.

Children are taught the exclusive use of the tooth brush, that cups and glasses (whatever the bacteriologist may say) are clean after being dipped in soap and water and rubbed with a cloth. They are now taught the exclusive use of their cups, but in May 1897 Mellins could advertise baby food in the *Illustrated London News* with a picture of big sister having a swig at the bottle. They are taught to eat bread with the fingers and meat (to the American left-handedly) with a fork. They are now taught, within a D.D.T. democracy, to make war on flies; but in an *Illustrated London News* of April 1895 Peek Frean and Co. advertised nursery biscuits with a picture of a child swotting a fly with a spoon. They are taught, in a rabies-free country, that dogs are nice and may be touched: 'You put out your hand steadily and the dog smells if you are friendly.'

[1] M. Mead (ed.), *Cultural Patterns and Technical Change* (U.N.E.S.C.O. 1955), p. 80. [2] *Ibid.* p. 72. [3] *Ibid.* p. 80.

Food avoidance

Children come to learn that some foods are forbidden. The English child avoids fungi and berries that are in fact edible—as the Austrian forest child is taught—and he is incapable of regarding the fox, squirrel, stoat, rat or horse as meat; but he is taught to like the kidneys and abhor the lungs of animals slaughtered for meat—the exact opposite of the German child.

Body contact

Habits of body contact are taught; kissing and where to kiss, the touching of sibs, parents, relatives and strangers, where to touch and where not to touch. Boys are taught differently from girls, so that in Britain no one is surprised to see women embrace or walk arm in arm; but the British are shy when European men embrace, and surprised to see African men link fingers.

Habits of body stance are taught: 'sit up, sit still, put your legs together' come automatically to the lips of British adults with growing daughters. The command is not quite the same to their growing sons—and were the parents conservative Muslim, they would say, 'Put your head down' to their daughter.

Sexual activity and restriction are taught. The incest taboos are safeguarded, girls are taught to be 'attractive', boys are taught to be 'manly'.

Evidence from the deprived child

All this leaves out of account the fact that people in association have an effect upon each other. Because this is so, the habit has arisen of calling the orphan, the institution child, among others, the 'Deprived Child'. That mere association has some effect is the theme of Bowlby.[1] Not all institutional children are warped, but it has long been recognised that such infants have high morbidity and death-rates, that they are late in walking and talking, and that they are often very polite and welcoming to adults. It is, of course,

---

[1] J. Bowlby, *Maternal Care and Mental Health* (W.H.O. 1951).

flattering when children are welcoming and polite. It is good for one's self-esteem to be welcomed in a children's home, in contrast with the reception from one's own children when all is well at home. When the parent returns in the evening, there is a nod of recognition, or at best an invitation to 'join in'; the children are fully occupied. If, when his key goes in the door, the response is running feet it means that for some reason—a quarrel, a catastrophe, a very special event—his arrival was awaited. What were the institution children doing before one's arrival? Nothing?

Children learn their attitude to strangers—varying from the approved outgoing response of babyhood to the withdrawn, 'Don't speak to strange men in the street, dear' of the adolescent girl, just as they acquire their attitude to authority. Is the policeman a public servant (on your side) or a bogeyman (on the other side)?

Not only does the institution child have to be introduced to money, the post office and buses for the same reasons that the town child has to be introduced to the cow, but he has also to be taught simple things, like body habits, and *meum* and *tuum*, which again are something of a problem for the town child in the country in respect of say, blackberries and apples, or public garden flowers and wild flowers. He has to be taught, too, something of incest taboos and other sexual behaviour. Even so, the effect of person upon person within an institution will be different from that of person upon person within a home. What those effects are it is not easy to say, but some of the links may be observed. Professor Illingworth says[1] that he has often been told by mothers in a four-bedded ward in a maternity unit that they do not awaken when a baby other than their own cries, but that they waken immediately when their own cries.

Dr Maclean had been Medical Superintendent of St Magnus Hospital for ten years or so. He had four sons—twelve years, ten years, seven years and four years. Finally a daughter was born to them. When the mother was asked on her first outing how she was and was her husband pleased, she told the questioner that over the years of marriage

---

[1] R. S. Illingworth, *B.M.J.* **1** (1955), 76.

the couple had settled to the classical pattern, where in the night the husband woke to the telephone and the wife to the children. She added, 'I really think he didn't hear the boys cry; but now he has a daughter, she has only to move in the night and he is out of bed and by her cot.'

Thus do we rear our sons—and daughters. On any one of these things and a host more there may be differences between the family and the neighbourhood norm, arising from any combination of the individual differences of the members of the family and the families' own environmental experience. Again these things come to bear ultimately upon the unique infant, and his response to these environmental factors depends ultimately upon his unique endowment.

This response in turn must, unless the child is to be in difficulty, conform more or less to the accepted patterns of behaviour not only in small things but in large, from eating to morals—and we are all subject to these pressures. Morals, codes of behaviour, may be held to be divinely inspired. It may be held that there is within us all a moral sense that distinguishes between right and wrong. Whatever view is taken, however, it is certain that children, to conform, must learn; there is general agreement that the earlier the child learns the better, and common acceptance that the home is the best place in which to learn.

CHAPTER IV

NEIGHBOURHOOD, SCHOOL AND HOME

SOCIAL PRESSURES OF THE NEIGHBOURHOOD

As the child grows his social horizon widens, and his culture is brought to him by an increasing number of people. The greatest widening takes place when he enters school. But no child will enter school without some experience of life outside his home, and none during the school years has his entire waking life divided between home and school. The neighbourhood exercises its pressure directly upon the child. Because of its importance in educational practice, and because of the increasing public assumption of its importance, the neighbourhood demand that children must play is examined here.

Play

One of the great changes in this country, as children have risen in public estimation, has been the increase in emphasis upon the child's right to play. It is assumed that the adult world is not suitable for children, and that children need special equipment—for the most part called toys—to occupy them. Conditions in industry a hundred years ago were generally accepted first as unsuitable for children and then for women, before they were regarded as altogether inhuman. Children were prohibited from working. Attitudes to schooling began to change, and less reliance was placed upon the adult's ability to teach and instruct the young and more upon the necessity of waiting for the physical and mental maturation of the young before instruction was undertaken. In middle-class homes, at least, parents came less and less to demand that their children be little adults. Parents became less certain of their own ability to inculcate the virtues which they wished for their child and fewer demands were made on children. This change occurred at a time when the number of servants employed was decreasing, and parents were compelled to be more directly concerned with their children. Because, too, the number of children which couples had born to them decreased, the children at home became more dependent upon adult company. The change occurred neither overnight nor universally. There are still many adults, for example, who had as children special, 'improving', provision for Sundays, when they were not allowed to play with everyday toys. There are, too, conservative clergy and church workers who are at least cautious towards, if not opposed to, week-day 'play-way' school methods penetrating to the Sunday school.

It has, however, become generally accepted as axiomatic and self-evident that children need to play. Many reasons are put forward: Herbert Spencer's excess of energy, William James's instinct to play, Professor Lazarus's aversion to being unoccupied, Karl Gros's biologically valuable preparation for life's more serious purposes, Stanley Hall's recapitulation of the history of the race, and Valentine's combination of these last two.[1] Many would subscribe to the late Sir Percy Nunn's statement:

> The impulse which drives the child along his life's course is not wholly absorbed by the activities necessary to maintain relations with the actual world. It urges him to multiply and enrich his experiences, to enlarge his soul by experiments in a thousand ways of life...the child's making-believe is a phenomenon of expansion, of growth. Unable through weakness and ignorance, to bend the stubborn reality of things to his will, to achieve his far-reaching purposes objectively, he employs the magic of making-believe, as Aladdin employed the genie of the lamp, to supply the means his ends demand, to make the world answer to his heart's desire.[2]

The nursery schools recognise the importance of play and, as we shall see, their basic notions have permeated the greater part of British educational provision. Children are in school, however, for only five hours of five days of the week, and for only forty weeks of the year. Work is prohibited, homes can rarely provide sufficient

[1] W. James, *Principles of Psychology* (London, 1901), vol. II, p. 427; C. W. Valentine, *The Psychology of Early Childhood* (London, 1942), ch. 9.
[2] *Education: Its Data and First Principles* (London, 1945), p. 92.

space for children to occupy themselves during their time out of school, and parents generally subscribe to the notion that children ought to play. There is in consequence public provision for children to play and every so often public concern about its suitability.

Facilities for play

Facilities for play are not as easily available for children as parents and the public now desire, and it is a common experience that without them children are troublesome. Mrs J. C. Ward found that about half the children living in flats and terraced houses in England play in the streets, and nearly ten per cent of those who live in flats never go out to play at all.[1] The percentage is probably higher among younger children living on or above the fourth floor.[2] There were 2440 children in the sample, and practically all said that the thing that they liked best to do was to play out of doors; but fifty-two per cent of them never went to the park and sixty-eight per cent had no access to a playground. Fewer mothers in the rural areas (twenty-six per cent) were satisfied with the play provision than mothers in the urban areas (thirty-eight per cent).

(1) *The cinema*

The largest activity among the children was the cinema clubs, and those who did not go at all were mostly the very young. A committee was appointed by the Home Secretary in 1948 to inquire into the attendance of children under sixteen at cinemas, and the survey was carried out by the Social Survey Division of the Central Office.[3] Children at modern schools go to the cinema more frequently than those at grammar schools, and those in the north of England more frequently than those in the south. In Scotland children go more frequently than elsewhere. The most common reason for disliking a film was that it was too frightening.

Cinema-going is a well-established habit among children. Children's cinema clubs affect only a minority of them, and mostly

[1] J. C. Ward, *Children out of School* (C.O.I. 1951).
[2] *Loneliness* (National Council of Social Service, London, 1957), p. 12.
[3] *The Times*, 9 November 1950.

the younger children. The chief reason for cinema-going appears to be the lack of alternative amusement, and it is suggested that children see films as a means of self-expression and should preferably be provided with other means.

(2) *The street*

The street is disapproved as a play-space, perhaps with too little reason, except for the traffic accident risk. Local authorities have powers to close streets to traffic, other than for delivery, so that they may be safe for children to play. There is something to be said, from the mother's point of view, for her young children playing near the open front door, more or less under supervision. As much household equipment as can prudently be commandeered is at hand, along with the child's own toys. Lavatory and water are near.

Older girls manage not unsatisfactorily if equipped with the basic chalk, ball and rope. Pavements are good for chalking, lamp-posts and railings suitable for swinging. A blank wall serves a purpose; so, too, does the curb. A sweet-shop opposite the blank wall gives her most that she can desire. Sweet-shops are open later than most shops; they give light on dark evenings, and provide a whole range of desirable objects for guessing games and forfeits.

Active boys find the street admirable for adventurous chasing and fighting games; but for football it is restrictive, and in cricket permits the bigger boy only the forward drive.

It is sometimes said that children do not play the traditional games. Observation in at least one working-class neighbourhood shows that the games are well known to contemporary children and are in fact played; but in more prosperous days these are not the only games they play. The top, marbles, grottoes, kites, skates, release, tip-cat, weak-horses, jimmy-nacker, knocking down ginger, daddy witch, five stones, cherry-hogs, conkers, dressing up, fireworks, guys, winter warmers, all turn up in the due season, along with hopscotch, the hundreds of guessing, divining games, methods of counting out, ball and skipping games (together with modernised versions of the rhymes), which are more popular with girls. These, especially the divining games and rituals, fade into adolescent beliefs as to what is and is not unlucky, 'signs', superstitions, and on into a folklore, surviving, especially among women, as general practitioners come to know, in connection with the children.

Children are noisy when they play, and it is a mark of a 'rough neighbourhood' that they do so in the street. This disapproval of the noise that children make is strong and widespread among British people.

(3) *Parks and playgrounds*

Local authorities have provided within their parks and in many smaller open spaces apparatus for children's play, and there is generally some supervision. The apparatus is for children under fourteen. It was welcomed in its day as an advance in the understanding of the needs of children. Today it is adversely criticised as being too rigid and restrictive in its possibilities. Children playing on bombed sites with bricks, old tyres, bedsteads, making shacks and lighting fires there, who had hitherto been regarded as troublesome, were seen in a new light when it became known that in Copenhagen and Minneapolis very similar material was being provided at some cost for 'disturbed' children. Beginning with the title of 'junk playgrounds', when secure in their place in British educational thought they became 'adventure playgrounds'. Voluntary societies have sponsored these playgrounds. One is described in *Social Work* (August 1953). In December of that year the Kensington Borough Council closed their playground at Ifield Road, after an expenditure of £3970, because it was 'too rough'. In April 1956 the *Times Educational Supplement* had a long illustrated article on an adventure playground in Grimsby.[1] Local authorities, including the London County Council, are cautiously making their playgrounds 'freer' and moving towards this type of provision.

[1] *Shanty Town*, a Report available from 29 Heneage Road, Grimsby (Grimsby, 1957).

School playgrounds are open after school and some in the school holidays as 'play-centres'. Often the school hall is available, too. Some organised games are played.

(4) *Organised groups*

In most areas churches, community centres and missions provide recreational play. Some of the groups—the Scouts, Boys' Brigade, Church Lads' Brigade—are uniformed.

Public concern with children's play is roughly no older than the century itself. Parents' axioms and self-evident assumptions about children have, for the most part, changed over those years. The changes must be understood if the doctor is to be aware of at least some of the factors that may be involved in difficulties as between home, neighbourhood and school, and for that purpose he must look for the concepts upon which these changes are based.

SOCIAL PRESSURES OF SCHOOL

General

It has, of course, long been recognised that schools are powerful forces for moulding children. Whatever the educational ideas and ideals of the school, there are also other important forces bearing down upon the children there. Some of these forces arise inevitably from the mere aggregation of the young under the care of the older.

Parents are sometimes first aware of speech changes—of a new accent (approved or disapproved), vocabulary or language. Children pick up two ways of speaking at school: the public one for staff and in class, and the more private one for conversation with contemporaries. Most British people go through life with at least three different ways of speaking: to superiors, to equals, and to the family circle.

Very soon it becomes clear to parents that children at school have learnt new ways of standing, new ways of moving their bodies and new standards of hygiene. These may be approved or disapproved.

Sometimes there is a deliberately sought culture conflict on the part of the schools, who support their own concept of their civilising mission; sometimes it is sought by parents who wish to advance their child. Sometimes the demands of either, but especially the school, may set quite unrealisable standards of child care.

Children at school are taught, like most young animals, to protect themselves against common dangers. Road drill, methods of disinfection and the accepted ways of body care are taught there.

Children, like puppies, must be exercised. As more and more interest is concentrated on the child and as the towns grow, the exercise of the young becomes more conscious and expensive. It ranges from the remedial, which is highly skilled and calls for individual attention, through the preventive, in carefully planned gymnasia, to games. This last can indeed be expensive in built-up areas, where land may cost £10,000 an acre; it costs far more for boys to kick a football about in Stepney than on the outskirts of Windsor. Children, like puppies, will take exercise somehow. They can in so doing make themselves an intolerable nuisance in towns, and even then fail to obtain the amount they need.

It is wasteful to try to teach a child who cannot pay attention because he is too ill, hungry, cold or tired. When compulsory education was first introduced in the 1870's, the condition of the children who were compelled to come in was such that, to the teaching staff at least, these observations were obvious. Some thirty years later (1900), in the interests of the children's education, means were provided for medical care of children, clothing and feeding. The *Report of the Interdepartmental Committee on Physical Deterioration*[1] and the *Report of the Interdepartmental Committee on Medical Inspection and Feeding of Children*[2] had revealed to an already awakened public the need for action. There were by 1884 sufficient medical officers in schools for them to form an association for promoting school hygiene. In 1890, the London School Board appointed a Medical Officer. The 1907 Act provided for systematic inspection and empowered local authorities to provide certain

[1] H.M.S.O. 1904.   [2] H.M.S.O. 1905.

forms of treatment, subject to the Board's consent. In 1918 local authorities were required to provide specified forms of treatment. The medical provision has, of course, burgeoned. Boot clubs used to be a regular feature of the old elementary schools. There is little need for them today. The feeding of 'necessitous' children remains. It was one of the intentions of post-war reform that every school child should be provided with a free and substantial mid-day meal. This never came about. About half the children attending maintained schools in England and Wales took the school dinner, and all but a very few paid for it.[1] In 1934 the milk-in-schools scheme was introduced and since 1946 the milk has been free. Less has been done about sleeping. In nursery schools and nursery classes it is usual for the children to rest in the afternoon. In 1914, Sir Cyril Burt then psychologist to the London County Council, reported that senior girls in a poor neighbourhood would do better at school subjects if they rested for part of each school day.[2]

Children learn manners at school—bad or good. There is a tendency for discussions on manners to become sententious. Manners are found everywhere, however, and not only in man. Man expects 'good manners' from the animals which associate with him. Before one puts one's small daughter across a pony for the first time one needs assurance that the pony has good manners— and what one asks of the pony is the same as one asks of man. Manners are linked with the common culture of a people, and, together with the philosophical and moral outlook, aspirations, and religion, are acquired at school.

Finally, children are taught to fend for themselves. Some things are consciously taught: reading, writing and arithmetic, a trade or skill; but some less explicitly: obedience, initiative, 'playing fair', looking after one's own interests and standing up for oneself—and when to pursue one of these and not the other. There is bound to be some vocational training, and with it, whether recognised as such or not, some vocational guidance.

[1] *School Meals Service*, Report of an enquiry into the working of the School Meals Service, 1955/56 (H.M.S.O. 1956).
[2] Sir C. Burt, *The Backward Child* (London, 1937), p. 125.

Educational objects

In the nursery school, the object is to assist the child to develop as a social being, rather than to sit him down and teach him, say, to read. The object is twofold: to help him to get along with other people, contemporaries and adults, as an independent individual, and to get him ready for learning. It sometimes happens that musical parents are so keen to teach their child music that he sheers off it for life. The nursery school tries to avoid that mistake: it does not deny the child who is ready the opportunity to learn to read, but it prefers to err on the side of caution to be assured that the child sees the point of reading.

Father on two nights running had missed the nightly story for Jo, for the simple reason that Father had his living to earn and twice running he had to stay late at work. 'Dad's hopeless, Mum', said Jo, sitting up in bed with the book in his hands. 'We'll never get on with this story unless I do it myself.'

The nursery school outlook is based upon the teaching of Froebel and Montessori; that outlook is common now in schools for children of all ages, and must therefore be understood.

Froebel

Although Froebel may be thought of almost exclusively in connexion with the pre-school child, neither his own thinking nor his influence have ended there. He was born in Thuringia in 1782. He called his schools children's gardens: *Kindergarten*. He, like many southern Germans, thought of children as plants, which grow according to laws inherent in their own nature and that the teacher's job is much the same as the gardener's: to provide the environment in which the child's abilities may unfold, secure from bad influences. He placed emphasis upon the importance of learning by doing and saw the early years of development as of pre-eminent importance. He saw, too, the interdependence of living things. He was critical of the methods of Pestalozzi, whom he regarded as placing too much emphasis on instruction, learning by rote and piecemeal—without sufficient regard to the integration of different subjects.

Froebel's ideas were part of the German Liberal movement destroyed in 1848. His school was suppressed then, but his ideas have spread and become incorporated in many theories and practices, including that of 'the child-centred school'. Much educational practice is based upon the concept that children are good—that if they are permitted to flower freely all will be well, and conversely that all evil is environmental.

The analogy appears to be that there is a notional perfect shape for flowers—and thus for children; but it is not pressed to the point where all flowers and children must be standardised, though this might appear to follow. Nevertheless, each flower, each child, has its unique endowment which must attain its individual fulfilment.

A good deal of nursery-school activity may be make-believe and fantasy. 'Pretend' is a word commonly in use, and make-believe is imaginative and 'good'. A notion associated with this outlook is that what the infant or child wants is good for him: his impulses are not dangerous or evil; the parents and teachers perform their function if they are permissive towards him. There is no need to send someone to see what Johnny is doing and to tell him not to. Johnny merely needs the opportunity to be good and he will be so.

An older school

Although Froebel's teachings have had a great vogue in Britain and in the United States, they do not commend themselves to all British parents. Some parents, loving their children, seek to give them a discipline which, they believe, will serve them well in life. Some parents may value what others have come to think of as 'old-fashioned'; and some schoolmasters will readily subscribe to these values and willingly educate children as their parents wish. Froebel's ideas do not commend themselves to those who believe that children are born in sin, and that it is only by the greatest care and regulation that the child can come to live the good life; that only by complete obedience and submission the child may be protected from the sin and evil inherent in his nature. Wesley, for example, planned every minute of the day for children at his school, Kingswood, for the devil finds occupation for idle hands; his school was to be no garden but a vigorous training ground of instruction. Education was not to be so much a 'leading out' as a 'putting in'. 'Induction' rather than 'education', it has been said. Some people will remember Aldous Huxley's 'Passively with his forty or fifty dissimilar and unique companions, he sits at his desk while the teacher pumps and mechanically repumps information into his mental receptacle', and his quotations of: 'Ram it in, ram it in! Children's heads are hollow, Ram it in, ram it in! Still there's more to follow.'[1]

Few schoolmasters today, however, would be pleased to read the last two sentences in a letter concerning the prep-school near Kensington Gardens which is mentioned in *Peter Pan*: 'I learnt more there in a short time than before or since, and always under duress. I never spent a day without the dread of what Milky would say or do to one who was in his eyes perhaps more than any other "a blithering little idiot".'[2] In an article concerning the school, the concluding sentences are:

At the end of my days a fearful thing happened to the school. An unexpected exodus of talented boys left me suddenly and all unworthily as its Head. I felt my position keenly. Nervously I took my place and Wilkinson entered the class room and glared.

'Not long ago', he remarked pleasantly, 'Shaw-Stewart sat there;[3] and now'—he pointed towards me the finger of denunciation—'This.'

The remark was indeed just. I would be the last to deny it. Yet it hurt quite a lot at the time. Odd that such a trifling wound can still rankle after a lapse of more than half a century.[4]

Schools, everywhere in Britain, are more easy-going places than, say, half a century ago. Those changes occurred first with the youngest children and were propagated most effectively in the schools of the local education authorities, for practically all their teachers, unlike those of the independent schools, are trained.

Instruction has for long been thought of as an unworthy pursuit in the universities of Britain; it has fallen into disfavour among the

---

[1] A. Huxley, *Proper Studies* (London, 1927), p. 97.
[2] *The Times*, 27 August 1956.
[3] The reference is probably to Patrick Shaw-Stewart (born 1888), a Fellow of All Souls, who joined the R.N.V.R. and was killled in action, 30 December 1917.
[4] *The Times*, 20 August 1956.

young at school. It survives, as something worthy of pursuit, at the top of the secondary and especially the grammar schools. It is a matter of contention between some parents and some teachers as to whether it has its place at the top of the primary school (see p. 173).

The differences in educational theories is well illustrated in the matter of handedness. Is the child to be taught to use his right hand? The old school says Yes and the newer No—and the newer attitude found its way to the home, so that children were, for example, allowed to eat 'left-handed'.

Shortly, it may be said that man has two hands, ordinarily he uses them together, the one for the coarser movement, the other for the finer one.[1] In some people the difference is very marked. If the movements are to be 'fine', it is clearly of advantage to train the appropriate hand, and if a child is compelled to perform movements with the 'coarser' hand which he may be able only just to achieve with his 'finer' one, the child may well run into difficulties. Two broad views may be taken. Conformity is important: the child's standard of writing may be lower with his right hand than his left, but it is preferable that he should conform. Alternatively, the individual is important: the child must write as well as possible and he must use his 'better' hand. There are all sorts of combinations of these views, and the point of decision for the individual child may be made anywhere between them.

Curious inconsistencies may be observed when the notion entered the dining-room. When the British use a knife and fork, the finer movement—conveying the food to the mouth—is done by the left hand. Seldom, if ever, are British children found who do not subscribe to this; yet the dominantly right-handed would probably prefer to do otherwise. Here custom is powerful. It is done because it is the British way, and not, for example, the Muslim way (where it is bad manners to convey food to the mouth with the left hand). This is not the way among the Americans, who use primarily only one instrument, putting down the knife to use the fork in the right hand. The right hand is used for the finer

[1] For a summary of views on handedness, together with foot, ear and eye preferences, see M. M. Clark, *Left-handedness* (London, 1957).

movement with spoon and fork. Sometimes British children are allowed to reverse the instruments. The right hand is used by the British when there is only one instrument—and it is here that the individual may now have choice. Even so, it is much rarer to find British children who are permitted to convey full cups of liquid to their mouths by their left hands.

An interesting sidelight is sometimes found on hand and eye dominance and its training in cricket. A boy has been taught to bat, right-handed—and he is not very good: he bowls left-handed. A left-handed bowler is much less of a nuisance than a left-handed batsman! A boy who is 'not very good at cricket' may take up tennis and like it and be good at it. If he holds his racquet in his left hand, a basic reason for his preference may be indicated, and a case may be made that a cricketer has been lost or spoiled. The older school might well maintain that, for a team game, the left-hander is worth his place only if he is outstanding and, if that is the case, he will 'come through' on his own.

Montessori

Some of the ideas of the late Dr Maria Montessori have been absorbed into educational practice; but her ideas have, on the whole, been less well received than more permissive ones in Britain.

Montessori was the first woman medical graduate of the University of Rome (1895). Her interest early turned to the mentally defective and their training. She was impressed by the laborious concentration of some defectives. She understood their need to apprehend the physical world, and she began to assist them by putting in their way finely graded apparatus by which their 'senses' might be trained. She went back to the work of Edouard Seguin, whose form-board finds its place to this day in psychological testing. She realised that defectives cannot be made to sit still: they cannot be trained after their interest has flagged. She developed the idea of 'controlled activity'. From the restricted range prescribed by the apparatus the child may choose his occupation, pursue it at his own pace, with the minimum interference from the teacher and abandon it when interest flags. She saw her defectives gaining a new 'freedom through discipline'. She noticed, too, the same 'work' factor in normal children's 'play'. She brought a new outlook to the understanding of the defective, and when her attention moved to the normal child, her ideas again transformed the school-room. The insistence on remaining quiet and still disappeared, and with it the system of rewards and punishments. The teacher's role was no longer to interfere: within the controlled environment, 'controlled activity' is possible. Her sense training of the defectives was necessarily manual. Her apparatus became a major part of the controlled environment, and a new stress was put upon manual activities at the expense of intellectual and imaginative activities.

'Pretending', fairy stories, and imaginative activities were, if not forbidden, at least discouraged. The child was to be corrected and brought back to 'reality'. Montessori's controlled environment, and especially her plain apparatus, most British educationalists would regard as anyhow restrictive and discouraging not only to imaginative play but also to creative play and to the exploration of colour and form. The late Sir Percy Nunn has said:

The Froebelians, believing that play has great educational value, encourage the child to make-believe because they think he cannot play without doing so. The Montessorians, who regard making-believe as frivolous and a form of untruth, are driven for the same reason to dispute the educational value of play.... Froebelian practice errs where it introduces making-believe gratuitously,...and the Montessorians err in refusing that aid where it would serve to widen the child's range of serious interests and achievements.[1]

Her system was warmly received by Mussolini, who perceived the essentially authoritarian nature of her outlook and the emphasis in her training upon conformity and adjustment. Her schools were, however, suppressed in 1936 in Italy and Germany.

Montessori came to realise that her system logically required her to start at birth, with the mother and her infant, and it would appear that the infant and toddler must be in the constant company of women able to provide the necessary stimuli.

[1] *Op. cit.*

HOME AND SCHOOL

Parents are not always aware of the educational outlook of the school to which they send their children, and may, unwittingly, compel their child to submit to a way of life there basically different from that of their home. Parents' choice of a school is often the end result of many considerations, not all explicit and not all of them would necessarily impress the observer as necessary and important. Apart from the basic notions—whether they really believe children to be essentially good or bad, or whether they think they should be liberated or controlled—parents cannot be expected to be clear about what they ask their child to acquire at school. Very generally, however, their hopes cluster around two heads: that he or she will be economically self-supporting and socially acceptable. Schools differ, however, in two main ways in the methods with which they achieve their objects. Roughly, the difference is between traditional schools and more modern ones. Education in the past has been thought of as essentially theoretical, best taught in the study, laboratory or class-room, that is, extrinsically. Modern thought is more practical, and looks much more to education 'on the job'—that is, intrinsically.

The problem is posed as soon as the parents ask where a child is to be educated and what he is to be taught. Is he old enough for school? They may think of their child as having hitherto been running about and 'learning nothing', and being now mature enough to be taken from his environment to be educated outside—extrinsically: put into the day school behind high brick walls with windows so high that no one can see out or in, and there taught things which some may say 'are no use to him'. He may be sent into the country, where most of the socially approved schools can be found, and taught there subjects of no direct use, say Latin and Greek. He may then be sent to a residential university, there to be prepared at the University for the law, his training will not be immediately practical, just as his engineering would be theoretical rather than practical.

A different view is to regard the small child at home as learning every minute of the day, learning about the way to do things. The girl learns at her mother's side to run the home, to bake, to mend, to shop, to negotiate; the boy learns his father's skills, skills from his contemporaries, skills from other people, until he is bound apprentice and he comes to learn on the job. Education is essentially practical, to do with everyday life and to be learnt on the job. It is intrinsic.

These two ideas are different from those of Froebel and of Montessori, and they relate themselves to their ideas in different ways. Speaking generally, just as Froebelian ideas have spread in Britain and have adapted themselves to the British way of life, so too has the tendency grown to make education and schooling more intrinsic. Arithmetic, by itself, is theoretical. Playing shops is something children like to do; and the rules of arithmetic will turn up when playing shops, along with a hundred other things. It is *playing shops*, however, and an illustration of the interconnection of things in life. The child may play at shops at school: but if he liked it so much as to want to do the real thing, out of school, the Law may be after the adult who permitted it, and the educationalists disapprove.

School buildings have changed in design. At the beginning of the century, among the essential things in a working-class area were a high brick wall and solid gates. The world could be shut out. Today there is no high brick wall. Railings there may be, but the school can be seen from the street and the street from the school. Moreover, there are large windows to the ground in the classrooms, opening not on to a cloister, but on to the street. The world is brought to the classroom, the classroom is in the world. Not everybody approves. Two elderly Bavarian Catholic priests, both teachers, came to this country to visit newly built schools. At the first glance at their first school, their reaction was immediate. Both said, in effect, 'I don't like it: there is no privacy. You can't *teach* in that.'

The permissive approach

There is fair certainty among British parents that manners can be explicitly taught only in part, and that they are largely acquired by processes which are not understood. Schoolmasters—especially

headmasters—set great store by the ability of their school to introduce boys to the values cherished by the British at large. This gives
comfort to parents who live within a swiftly moving culture and
are themselves uncertain of how to teach truth, beauty and goodness to their children—and worried because they value these things
and love their children. Few parents can say that they know exactly
how to teach, not the children next door, but their own children,
the difference between right and wrong, about love, morals and
God. Now if this is true of parents generally, schoolmasters themselves cannot altogether escape the same anxieties, and the notion
that the child is essentially good provides the theoretical justification
for 'letting the child decide'. Catholic and Jewish thought cannot
subscribe to this.

One result of this permissive approach to the child has been, says
K. Soddy, that in Britain considerable emphasis is laid upon the
moral development of young children, upon the inculcation of a
sense of duty and upon personal responsibility. From a very early
age children may be required to make decisions, and not only to do
this but to make the 'right' decision for the 'right' reasons. He
sees a dilemma between inculcating a sense of responsibility and
making the child too anxious.[1]

He also makes it clear that he is comparing this situation with that
of a child reared in a society where 'no one questions the detailed
regulation of forms of behaviour and it is, therefore, unlikely that
the child will develop any notion that there might exist a possibility
of a choice between alternative courses of behaviour, much less any
choice between alternative moral attitudes'. He raises two important questions in relation to education: culture conflict and the
degree of regulation. The mere fact that 'there might exist a
possibility of a choice between alternative courses of behaviour' is
present for the Muslim family, for example, in India, if the family
across the road is Hindu. The situation is at first simple: I am right
and he is wrong. Difficulties begin with the questioning: Is he
altogether wrong, am I altogether right? Then what to teach the

---

[1] K. Soddy, 'Mental Health and the Upbringing of Small Children' in
Family, Mental Health and the State (W.H.O., Pt. 2, 1955), p. 22.

child becomes a painful, anxious question. How this may arise and whether the effect will be damaging is not understood. Whereas formerly it had been assumed that the gradual process of change brought fewer difficulties, the experience of the war and post-war years when, especially in the Pacific, peoples had their way of life overturned by the sudden and forceful impact of mainly American ways, has led to the questioning of this assumption. In her reassessment of the Manus in 1953, after twenty-five years, Margaret Mead puts forward the possibility that the swiftness of the changes was an essential element in their success.[1]

The child in Britain is exposed to culture conflict, between the generations (p. 11), between school and home (p. 52), and, from the very fact of tolerance, between religion and religion and political party and political party. The problem is not a new one in Britain and today, at a guess, is not as severe for the greater number of the educated as it was in the days when Mrs Humphry Ward wrote *Robert Elsmere*, when the whole basis of life was being questioned by the scientists, and the Christian faith was being subjected to the higher criticism. It certainly does not exist in Britain in so severe a form as it did for families reared between the wars in Germany.

Culture conflict does, however, exist in Britain and presents itself as an individual and family problem; but it is probably subordinate to the problems which arise from variation in the degree of regulation of the child, particularly if there are marked differences between school and home.

We have seen that traditional British schooling, Froebelian, and Montessorian methods differ in the amount and way of regulating and controlling the child. We have seen that the liberating Froebelian ideas may ally themselves with the trend to teach 'on the job'. The Froebelian liberating outlook may, it has been suggested, provide a theoretical basis for 'letting the child decide' not only whether to play the flute or the violin but whether there is or is not a God. It is as well to notice that these ideas may be in fundamental conflict with the moral and religious outlook of the home.

[1] M. Mead, *New Lives for Old* (London, 1956).

Permissive approach and the home

It would be possible to put in some rough order the religions found in Europe and America according to their belief about the character of man. At one extreme he would be considered utterly foolish, at the other undoubtedly good. The more foolish man is, the more important it becomes for the wise or the inspired to provide for and legislate for man's affairs. Only thus will human life be possible. The more naturally good man is, the more important it is to liberate him and to allow him to develop.

Orthodox Jewry provides the most extreme example, for most Europeans, of the highly regulated religions, where the whole day and year is minutely regulated, and wise men, always and consciously moving slowly and cautiously, provide for the changing world. The Christian religions are less desirous of minute regulation. Jesus said that two commandments were enough—but clearly the Catholic Church places much more emphasis upon (without irreverence) 'Father knowing best' than, for example, the Society of Friends, who emphasise the over-riding importance of the individual conscience and the 'inner light'. The further one moves away from the Catholic position to that of the Society of Friends, the further does the status of the priest decline until he finally disappears.

It is possible for some parents to argue from the premise of man's foolishness that the methods of psychotherapy and those of the more modern teachers are anarchical. That argument can be sustained without necessarily condemning the objects of both as undesirable. Psychotherapeutic method and modern educational method have, however, both found increasing favour among people in Britain.

An incidental consequence of the increasing favour of the permissive factor in modern education and in psychotherapy is the popular misrepresentation of Freud's teaching. Freud taught that anxiety and fear are civilising forces, whereas he is thought to have taught that all frustration is bad. Another consequence is to think of Adler's teaching as a popular explanation of intolerable behaviour in others and not as a description of the positive force that leads to the exercise of gifts and talents.

The older and newer

The amount of emphasis laid upon the inculcation of a sense of duty and of personal responsibility varies within schools as much as it does within homes, and conflict may arise, apart from religion, between the teaching of the school in these matters and the households of farmers, shopkeepers, costers, clergymen, policemen, C.P.O.'s and R.S.M.'s—and this is a factor to be taken into account when considering the child at school.[1] At the back of a good deal of thinking about schools there is the assumption that somewhere, if we can only hit on it, there must be the correct way to run a school. Discover it, provide it, and all will be well.

The sort of schools produced and what is taught there is largely dependent upon the aims and ideals of society. The conscious planning of education to make a certain type of product does not come easily to the British, but they achieved something very like it with adolescents and young men between 1939 and 1945. If there is a single organised system of ideals, be it Fascism, Communism or Catholicism, it is perhaps possible to devise a system of education which will produce, with the minimum of casualties, the required types with the approved outlook. There can be a coherent theory of education, and the problem of classifying becomes merely one of placing the individual child in his appropriate niche in the single system.

The British have never had a single organised system of ideals (except for the few years of war). But perhaps after all they have: the ideal that there is room for everyone, whatever their way of life, their ideas and ideals. There must, therefore, be all sorts and varieties

---

[1] N. Kent and D. Russell Davies show that eight-year-old children from primary schools whom they investigated did measurably better on the Binet test when they came from 'demanding homes' than when they came from homes classified as 'normal', 'over-anxious' or 'unconcerned' (*Brit. J. Med. Psychol.* 30 (1957), 27).

of schools to achieve this very ideal, and many of the schools will, of necessity, be somewhat uncertain about their purpose.

A glance over history reminds us that the most vital and effective systems of education have envisaged their objectives quite concretely, in terms of personal qualities and social situations. Spartan, Feudal, Jesuit, Nazi, Communist educations have had this in common, they knew what they wanted to do and believed in it. By contrast, education in the liberal democracies is distressingly nebulous in its aims.[1]

'All parents who can afford it should send their children to public schools', or 'the only decent form of education is to be found in the progressive schools'—these statements are sheer projection (see p. 92). What the physician does with his own children is (in Britain) entirely between him, his income and his ideals. When he comes to consider the schooling of a patient, he is concerned first with his patient, then the patient's family, their ideas and ideals, and how best the patient's interests can be met within the context. If the father is in the diplomatic service and the mother is an admiral's daughter, the fact that their son is an unhappy failure at his public school is not necessarily resolved by sending him to a progressive school run by a leftish proprietor, and patronised by parents who are modern artists. The fundamental differences in outlook between home and school may or may not be relevant: these factors can be neglected, however, only at the gravest risk. A nice assessment of many factors is necessary. Children may do badly at a progressive school.

Robin and Roger were the sons of a parson and his doctor wife. Both were sent to a progressive school. Robin, the elder, never settled down. He was not good with his hands and felt inferior because he had no manual talent. He was uneasy in the permissive atmosphere. He became argumentative and obstructive. He was taken away and sent to an orthodox day school. He settled into the routine quickly, within a year caught up with the school-work, and showed thereafter marked ability in the classics.

Roger had no ability with his hands either but he was happy at school and after a contented and idle year in the permissive atmosphere began to show interests similar to his brother's. Facilities were available for him and he followed his brother to the university to read classics.

[1] M. V. C. Jeffreys, *Glaucon* (London, 1950), p. 61.

CHAPTER V

DISCIPLINE AND THE CHILD

PUNISHMENT AND WELFARE

The doctor in practice seldom or never administers punishment; but the permitted sanctions at home, at school, and by society at large, may well have loomed large in the child's life before he is presented to the doctor.

Children, when they are troublesome to adults, are punished. The efficacy of punishment is considered sometimes to be in associating something unpleasant (punishment) with the forbidden act, sometimes in shaping the individual so that he avoids, perhaps mechanically, the act, or sometimes in removing from the individual the desire to perform it. Punishment comes from outside, and aims to change the individual.

There is another approach to the troublesome child. In this approach the disapproved behaviour is thought to arise from some organisational reason: therefore nothing has to be removed from the make-up of the individual, or shaped, or made unpleasant; the human endowment of the child, which is essentially good, has simply got 'mixed up', 'disturbed' or 'maladjusted'. As an extension, sometimes the environment has to be adjusted; an unusual pressure removed or lightened, or, because of a recognised disability in the child, a more common one modified.

The two views are conflicting. In everyday life both attitudes are often present in dealing with the child. It may be demanded, for example, that the child who steals be punished and that after punishment, or in the course of it, he be investigated for maladjustment. Children from infancy may be regarded from either viewpoint. In any event, there comes a time when a child must be regarded as responsible for his actions. When that point is reached, the adult expressions of disapproval of his action are no longer thought of as training and education, but as remedial, as re-training or re-education. It follows that the younger the child, the more rare the remedial process. A child is not assumed, in law, to know the difference between right and wrong until he is fourteen. Young children, then, those whose mental ability is no more than that of a child, and those who are mentally deranged, are not subjected to the remedial processes of either punishment or welfare: whatever is done is, supposedly, part of training and education.

Characteristics of punishment

Punishment is the penalty for wrong-doing, for offending against ethics, laws, mores or folkways. It may be an individual who inflicts it, but he does so as the representative of a group. At least five characteristics of punishment are to be noted.

(1) Retribution

Punishment may be retributive: the boy must learn that inevitably, mechanically, if he has offended against parents or school, brought harm, disgrace, or ill-repute to them, punishment will come to him. In the wider community, similar ideas are built up: he who sins against God or injures the community is punished. Comforting (or frightening, depending upon the point of view) ideas are built up on this notion, like 'murder will out' although the evidence is that in England and Wales the odds of detection are not more than even.

(2) Deterrence

Punishment is also deterrent, aiming either by its severity, or, much more effectively, by its certainty, at preventing the recurrence of the wrong-doing either in the individual or in others or in both. The constant association of pain or unpleasantness with an act or an object is deterrent: this is how children learn about fire, cattle about electrified wires.

(3) Reformation

Punishment may be reformative: it will teach a lesson, by reinforcing the principles which have been already taught or breaking the resistance which may have grown up against their observance.

The child must do as he is told; he must not challenge authority; he must not be allowed to get away with that. Children will challenge the authority of the new or young teacher, and at home, that of an older sib or an aunt, and, sometimes, that of their parents. Sometimes associated with reformation is the notion of restitution: that damage must be made good, what has been taken must be replaced.

(4) *Example*

So far, punishment has been regarded as something brought to bear upon the individual, because of his individual wrong-doing: he is threatened, penalised by the group upon which he himself is dependent, and at the worst, he may be removed from the group—expelled from school, sent away to school, or with adults (formerly banished and later transported) sent to prison or hanged. Punishment is between society and the culprit. Exemplary punishment is between society and the culprit. Exemplary punishment, however, shows another aspect. For example, smoking has been going on at a school for a long time and one boy is caught. He may be punished for the foregoing reasons and he may further be punished 'to make an example of him'—to teach a lesson to all those who are undiscovered but known to exist. There may well be contained in this aspect of punishment the notion that wrong-doing known to a society and unpunished causes a dangerous frustration of emotion: if punishment cannot be brought to all offenders, it must necessarily be vented with particular violence on the one who is caught—as with the traditional whipping-boy. Some schoolmasters and parents use children in a way uncommonly like whipping-boys who bear the whole burden of what in another vocabulary is called the displacement of affect. Perhaps the illegitimate child is the whipping-boy in place of his sinful parents. The accepted use of this aspect of punishment is its effect upon the subgroup of which the culprit is a member. Now it is possible for the punishment to strengthen the loyalties of the subgroup and for the culprit to return to it with an enhanced status. This happens today among male homosexuals, for example, where the group see no way of finding their ordered place in society and may well come to recognise their rejection and reinforce their own loyalties. This defeats the object of punishment, which is to retain the individual within the proper ordinations within society. Murder, rape, stealing, arson, are all offences punishable within a society. To the external enemies of society, however, fire and sword is taken, and the spoils of war are lawful: actions which are crimes within a society cease to be crimes when committed against a hostile group.

(5) Group punishment

Punishment may be inflicted upon a whole group, because within it are individuals who have injured society but are inaccessible, unidentifiable or protected by the whole group; and therefore in the interest of order, because punishment must be delivered, the whole group is punished. When at school 'no one will own up', a whole class is sometimes punished, and a village which will not deliver up its law-breakers may be fined corporately. The notion appears to be that the pain of punishment will make the individuals of the group turn against the individual wrong-doer and mete out punishment themselves, and will thus prevent a recurrence of the offence. The principle is one old-established in English justice and surviving in the finding of sureties. Its efficacy depends in part upon the severity of the punishment, and in part on the degree of attachment or regard of the group to the punisher as opposed to the culprit. The effect may simply be to bring about war between the group and the punisher.

The efficacy of punishment, except group punishment, depends upon the strength of the attachment between punisher and culprit: where the attachment is strong, punishment is effective and rarely necessary; where the attachment is weak, punishment merely reinforces the culprit's sense of disorganisation and evokes his hostility.

Punishment—a social act

The awarding of punishment is therefore a responsible social act. Now some people enjoy responsibility a great deal more than others, but to play the part of the upholder of right is to many an attractive role, and the infliction of punishment, especially when the crime has been brutal, is particularly satisfying; this satisfaction may be seen in the judge on the bench, the administrator within his territory, the schoolmaster with his class, the parents with their child—and children with children.

Were each one of us sure of all our duties to all our loyalties and how those loyalties were related one to the other, and were we all convinced in both mind and heart of the rightness of the world, the logic of punishment would be clear and certain and, more, there would probably be no place for punishment, for each one would be guided by himself—by his conscience. In a multi-purpose society, however, tolerant of conflicting moral, religious and political ideals and rapidly changing, the individual is often, perforce, faced with how to avoid censure and punishment, how to reconcile his own way of life with society as he finds it.

PUNISHMENT BY PARENTS

Parents and children may not only be guided by conscience, but also be painfully self-punishing. Many British parents will deny that they punish their children, or confess with shame that they have 'got mad' with their child and struck him. Sterner parental discipline does survive but there is public disapproval: beating, for example, at school is now almost entirely reserved for those who are sent to expensive and traditional boys' schools, and even there is less in vogue than formerly. Both the permissive and authoritarian parent (and school) are held within social bounds: a statement like 'their children do what they like' should rarely be taken literally, any more than should 'their children are punished for the slightest thing'. It this were so, both parents could certainly be charged, the one with neglect and the other with cruelty.

London working-class parents pacify their infants rather than punish them. The crying baby, whatever the current fashion of teaching may be, is picked up and perhaps fed. The rubber teat is called a pacifier. In small houses the need to keep the children quiet continues throughout childhood and pacification, particularly by food and sweets, is regular. Mothers may be observed—though they often deny it—slapping their toddlers. The punishment is a deterrent. The toddler must not touch—and the raised hand is slapped down and the child is told 'no'. As the child grows, mothers resort to shaking and thumping their children about the shoulders. Rarely do mothers smack about the face or buttocks. Canes can still be bought in village and working-class 'oil shops', but their use is rare and their purchase is an open confession of failure.

Mothers abandon corporal punishment by the time their children are twelve or so and rely for its administration, if necessary, upon father. The belt and slipper are the traditional instruments. Few fathers use them and the hullabaloo will announce the proceedings to all and sundry. Father is much more likely to clout the children in a fit of anger when he regards his wife as unable to control them and is finding them insufferable. The situation is to be explained in terms of the physical release of emotion, rather than of thought-out punishment. Parents, and especially mothers, threaten their children: 'Mummy won't love you if', 'Mummy will give you away if', 'The policeman will take you away if'. As the children grow, in some neighbourhoods and especially in London, mothers can rise to a sustained, poetic and surrealist abuse. In the course of her tirade against her twelve-year-old she may (1) reject him—tell him to go away, moving towards him; (2) offer physical punishment; (3) threaten corporal punishment from his father; (4) deprive him, say, of his picture money; (5) abuse him for any physical, mental, or temperamental characteristics which may occur to her; and (6) pacify him by giving him money to buy ice-cream, thus terminating the scene. The competent mother may achieve all this in a paragraph and convey to her child that temporarily she would prefer his room to his presence—and no more.

Parents deprive their children as a punishment of spending money, of food, of visits. Actual deprivation is moving towards the severer punishments, for with most parents actual deprivation defeats its object; it results in crying, whining, pleading children, and order has to be restored by some sort of pacification. For a child to take the deprivation without fuss implies a more authoritative discipline than is usually found, as does the most serious current punishment of sending to bed. Parents usually rely upon their tongues to deal with troublesome children. The most usual and effective and mildest is the loudest, when the mere volume of the parental voice is used like a physical assault and emotional release. English, with its finely graded vocabularies, is peculiarly suited to this form of discipline, for the volume can be strengthened with a word or two prohibited to children to use. The voice is in my observation an effective disciplinarian, the degree of effectiveness depending upon the attachment between parents and children.

The constant reiteration of complaint: 'Why do you do these things?', 'Why aren't you a good boy?', 'Why don't you behave like your brother?', is an admission of failure, ineffective and solidly disapproved. With their older children, Londoners, at any rate, are adept at the use of sarcasm, using it not only for punishment but also for the oblique discussion and illumination of family difficulties. Perhaps the greatest deprivation and punishment is to 'take no notice of him'. Then the attachment is threatened if not broken.

Parents, and particularly the older ones, are very much aware that discipline and punishment within the home have changed. Many working-class parents will volunteer that they were afraid of their fathers, mainly because of his unpredictable violence.

PUNISHMENT BY TEACHERS

Corporal punishment is retained in British schools and is regarded by the North American and European as an educational curiosity. One survey found that 89.2 per cent of teachers in British schools were of the opinion that it should be retained.[1] Its use, however, is strictly circumscribed by the local authorities, who usually restrict its execution to the headmaster, prescribing the amount, and arranging for a record to be kept and witnesses to be present, for there is always the risk that parents may have recourse to the courts.

[1] *Rewards and Punishments* (National Foundation for Educational Research, London, 1952).

73

But moderate chastisement may in law be inflicted not only by a parent upon his child but by a schoolmaster upon his scholars, and any parent who sends his child to school is presumed to give the teachers authority to administer reasonable corporal punishment. Only senior boys are struck on the buttocks; for some reason girls and younger boys are struck on the hand. In the independent schools beating is much less fashionable than it used to be. The arrangements, however, are much more informal there and any parent (and boy) knows that if the boy is sent to the school he may run the risk of beating. Girls' independent schools rarely, if ever, beat.

Substitute physical punishments are used in independent schools and in local authority ones—work on the school grounds, sweeping, cleaning up, cross-country running. Children are detailed to carry out monotonous tasks, such as the written repetition of a dictum like 'I must not talk in class', or of the Latin or Greek verbs. The punishment lies partly in the deprivation of leisure, partly in the laborious repetition. There is also reliance on the efficacy of repetition in learning, as there is when a child is told to 'do his work again'.

In many day schools, for obvious reasons, punishment after school hours is unpopular with the staff, and school breaks, lunch hours and games periods may be used.

Scoring systems for competition between groups of children—often called houses, whether the children board or not—combine both punishment and reward, and are approved because of the corporate nature of both aspects. The delinquent may serve the school society by cleaning up or sweeping; he runs the risk of public censure if he 'lets the side down' by losing points.

Teachers evolve their own informal systems of punishment within the classroom, both physical and verbal, calling upon any or all of the methods used by school and parents and reinforcing them sometimes by ridicule.

When the school is avowedly permissive, punishment may be altogether abandoned; but wrong-doing is not thereby abolished. Reasoning and the appeal to a better self may be used, so that the burden of correction is thrown upon the child himself. Some reorganisation of the environment may be undertaken to avoid a repetition of the wrong-doing. Violent behaviour may necessitate restraint but violence and deeply disapproved behaviour would be the subject of investigation and treatment; intractable behaviour would lead to removal from the school—an admission of failure. It is fair to add that similarly intractable and deeply disapproved behaviour would be punished by expulsion in more conservative schools, too. The parent, whatever his outlook, cannot have recourse to this remedy himself.

Finally, the fewer the regulations, that is, the more permissive the environment, the less the occasions for punishment. This is of course as true at home as at school. I discovered, to my dismay, that when sweets were rationed it was I and not my children who stole them. I gave the whole of my ration to my children and all the sweets were kept in a large stoppered jar in their playroom. The sweets were theirs—they helped themselves as they wanted them. Father had no sweets: all sweets belonged to the children. When father locked up at night and the children had been in bed some hours, he often helped himself. If anyone stole sweets, it was father. Speaking generally, the more permissive schools seek a discipline analogous to that of the home, relying upon a minimum of rules to observe and an adequately strong attachment between child and staff. The more traditional schools depend less upon methods usually associated with folkways and mores and rely more upon those associated with the law. Some of the punishments used—the group and exemplary ones for instance—though common in colonial administration and appearing occasionally in adult courts, as we shall see, are rare in the present-day treatment of juvenile delinquents.

PUNISHMENT BY SOCIETY AT JUVENILE COURTS

When children come into conflict with the law, they become subject to procedures, punishments and remedies different from those of schools—except for the partial similarity in the more traditional school—and different from those of home.

Children who are arrested must be kept separate from adults, except from the adult with whom they are jointly charged, at the police station and in the courts, and girls must be in the care of a woman. Children may have bail, like adults, unless the charge is homicide or some other grave crime, or unless it is necessary to remove him in his own interest from association with any reputed criminal or prostitute, or unless there is reason to believe that release would defeat the ends of justice. The child is detained separately from adults.

Practically all charges against children are heard in the juvenile courts. The exceptions are cases of homicide or cases in which a juvenile is charged with an adult. The right of a child over fourteen years to be tried by jury is rarely exercised.

Children before the courts fall into five groups.

(*a*) Children who are charged with an offence. The court may deal with the case—that is, find the child guilty or not guilty, except where the charge is homicide; then the court acts as examining magistrates and commits the child to trial (if appropriate) in the adult court.

(*b*) Children whose parents are charged with offences under the Education Act. The children are then dealt with as in need of care and protection.

(*c*) Children who are the subject of an Adoption Order (see p. 126).

(*d*) Children whose parents or guardian have submitted that they are beyond control.

(*e*) Children who are brought before the court as being in need of care and protection.

The juvenile court (established under the Children Act, 1908) must be separate from other courts, either sitting on a different day or in a different building. The Justices must be members of a panel of those who are specially qualified to deal with juvenile cases. Every juvenile court consists of not more than three Justices and includes one man and, if practicable, one woman. The chairman is nominated by the Secretary of State. The only persons who may be present are members and officers of the court, parties to the case, their solicitors and counsel, representatives of newspapers and such other persons whom the Court may authorise (generally students). The child's right to public trial is safeguarded by the press; but the publication of the child's name, address and photograph is forbidden. The child's appearance in court on some charges must be notified to the probation officer appointed to the court and to the local authority, so that the court may have available information about home surroundings, school record, health and character of the child, and, where appropriate, approved schools.

To assist the magistrates in deciding upon a proper course of action, there may be written reports from the local education authority, the probation officer, the children's officer, and any special information such as a medical or psychological report. They are bound to communicate to the parents anything in the report which influences them in their decision about the child.

No child under eight years of age can be guilty of an offence. For a child between the ages of eight and fourteen, the prosecution must prove not only that the child committed the offence but also that he had guilty knowledge that he was doing wrong. After the age of fourteen the child is deemed to have sufficient discretion to know the difference between right and wrong unless there is positive proof of mental derangement or imbecility.

The court must explain to the child the substance of the charge in simple language suitable to his age and understanding. He is entitled to assistance by way of free legal aid, in the same way as adults. In practice, however, it is far from easy to ensure that a child knows what is happening. When he is charged with an offence and pleads 'not guilty' (as he may be advised to do, perhaps contrary to his own inclination) difficulties occur over the oath. This is still retained in the juvenile court and the child is confronted with the choice of taking the oath and being cross-examined, making a statement, or saying nothing.

Remedies

It is not until after the child has been found guilty that remedy is considered. Punishment in the group sense is unknown in the juvenile court; punishment as example is rare as, too, is the purely deterrent one. The factor of retribution may often be discernible if not explicit, but the main intention of the court is that of reformation. Indeed, throughout the courts, both civil and criminal, the child's interests are always of paramount importance. After the finding of guilt the court is concerned more with the child's welfare than with his punishment. There is sometimes a conflict of interest between welfare and the administration of justice: the child may well be in need of services which the court can provide, but first a charge against him must be legally proved. This difficulty is not peculiar to juveniles: it occurs wherever welfare and justice are in partnership. One must be the dominant partner.

(1) *Discharge*

The child may be absolutely discharged if the court, having found the child guilty, is of the opinion that, having regard to the circumstances, including the nature of the offence and the character of the child, it is inexpedient to inflict punishment, and that a probation order is not appropriate. The child may be discharged subject to the condition that he does not commit another offence during a maximum period of twelve months.

(2) *Probation order*

A probation order may be made, the effect of which is that for a given period of time (not less than one and not more than three years) the child undertakes to be of good behaviour, to keep in touch with the probation officer, carry out his instructions and also undertake any special requirements of the order (usually referring to residence). Probation hostels are provided, and where they are available they give to adolescents a valuable opportunity to steady themselves away from home. There are approved lodgings which may be useful to give the probationers a substitute home for a shorter or longer period. Probation training homes exist which give an environment not dissimilar from an approved school. If the child fails to carry out the condition or commits another offence, he is liable to be sentenced for the offence in respect of which the order is made. The order is made, that is to say, for the child to 'prove' himself. The probation officer undertakes to advise and befriend the child. A supervision order is generally similar: it is used when the child is either beyond control or in need of care and protection. The difference in nomenclature is necessary, for the child, in these cases, has committed no offence.

(3) *Fines*

A child may be fined; so too may be the parents and guardians of a child who has committed an offence and damages or costs may also be recovered from them. Here the hope is that reformation will be achieved by the insistence upon restitution.

(4) *'Fit person' order*

A child may be committed to the care of a 'fit person'—whether a relative or not—who is willing to undertake the care of him, if the offence of which he has been found guilty is, in an adult, punishable by imprisonment. The order normally remains in force until the child is eighteen and the person to whose care a child is committed has, while the order is in force, the same rights and powers and is subject to the same liabilities in respect of his maintenance as if he were the parent. The local authority is deemed to be a fit person. The orders may, on the application of any person, be varied or revoked. Parents have a statutory duty to contribute to the maintenance of their children until they are sixteen years old.

(5) *Approved school*

A child over ten years of age (or younger, if there is no fit person of his own religious persuasion who is willing to undertake the care of him) may be committed to an approved school. If the child is under sixteen years of age at the time of the order to commit, it runs for three years. If he is over sixteen, then it runs until he is nineteen, or nineteen and a half if a new order is made. These schools are not part of the education system. They are schools approved by the Home Office as suitable for the industrial training and reformation of young delinquents: they are indeed the successors to the industrial schools and reformatories.

The schools are in three age categories: junior (ten to thirteen), intermediate (thirteen to fifteen), and senior (fifteen to seventeen). Children may be licensed—though this is exceptional in the first twelve months—to live with their parents or any named trustworthy and respectable person. After the expiry of the period of the order, the child is under the supervision of the school managers —if he has not attained the age of fifteen—until he is eighteen, or if over fifteen, for three years or until he attains the age of twenty-one. During the time of supervision the child may be recalled. A child on licence from an approved school may be taken into care by the local welfare authority if he has no home, or his home is thought to be unsatisfactory by the school managers. Some schools have their own hostels from which boys and girls go out to work before they are finally licensed and return home. A child who on the day of conviction is not less than fifteen but under twenty-one may be sent to Borstal training, which is for both boys and girls. The juvenile court commits the child to sessions for Borstal sentence.

(6) *Detention centre*

Since the war two new forms of punishment have been introduced; the detention centre and the attendance centre. These administer upon the retributive factor in punishment. The detention centre, according to the Home Office, is intended to give a 'short, sharp shock' to boys who have not yet developed a definitely anti-social attitude, but who need to be taught that the law cannot be defied with impunity. A boy may not be detained there unless he is over fourteen and under twenty-one and unless the court has considered every other method (except imprisonment) of dealing with him and is of the opinion that none of those methods is appropriate. Ordinarily a boy is sent there for three months, and the maximum period is six months.

(7) *Attendance centre*

The attendance centre is designed for the child over twelve who has not previously been sentenced to prison, borstal, detention centre, or approved school. He attends for not more than twelve hours, not more than once a day and at times that will not interfere with work or school.

(8) *Prison*

Children may still be sent to prison. A magistrates' court cannot impose imprisonment on any person under seventeen; but a court of assize or quarter sessions may impose imprisonment on persons over fifteen. When it does so, however, it must be of the opinion that no other method of dealing with him is appropriate, must take into account information concerning his physical and mental condition and must state the reason for its opinion that no other method of dealing with the boy is appropriate. These would be that the offender is of so unruly a character that no method of dealing with him, other than imprisonment, is appropriate, or that he is so depraved a character that he is not a fit person to be dealt with otherwise than by imprisonment.

Few today would imagine that a child sent to prison is likely to benefit by his experience there. But prison is the nearest society can now come to ridding itself of its failures: transportation or death were more thorough ways of removing them, but neither method is available today. In February 1953, at the West Kent Assizes, a boy of fifteen was jailed for five years. He had a record of 105 offences. He had absconded eight times from approved schools. In December 1952 he had been found guilty of housebreaking and 39 other cases were taken into consideration. In January he took from his mother's purse £6. 10s. The punishment may contain retributive, deterrent factors; but the attitude of the court is more likely to be despair.

(9) *Remand home*

The 'special reception' centre for children under twelve, the 'remand home' for children under seventeen and the 'remand centre' for those over seventeen (or over fourteen if unruly or depraved) are not, properly, places of punishment. Adults may be remanded (*remandare*—to send word back) that is, sent back to prison (old French *prisun*—the action of taking). Remanding in custody is used for the safe-keeping of the accused, for mental and physical investigation and, after a finding of guilt, may be used again for temporary safe-keeping and classification. If the child is found guilty of an offence which in an adult is punishable by imprisonment and the court considers that none of the other methods by which a case may be legally dealt with is suitable, the court may order the child to be committed to custody in a remand home for a period not exceeding one month.

(10) '*Beyond control*'

A parent or guardian or a local authority who has a child in care may prove to a juvenile court that they are unable to control the child. The court may send the juvenile to an approved school, or make a supervision order for the probation officer, or some other person appointed by the court for the purpose, to watch over him, or make a 'fit person' order for his care by a fit person.

(11) *Care and protection*

A child may be found to be in need of care and protection for three main reasons.

(*a*) He may have no parent or guardian, or a parent or guardian unfit to exercise care and guardianship or not exercising proper care and guardianship; be falling into bad associations, exposed to moral danger, or beyond control; or be ill-treated or neglected in a manner likely to cause him unnecessary suffering or injury to health.

(*b*) He may have suffered an offence involving bodily injury (including sexual offences), or be a member of a household where another child has suffered these injuries, or where a person has been convicted of these offences, or (if female) where a person has been convicted of incest.

(c) He may be a member of the family of a vagrant who prevents him from receiving efficient education.

Ingleby Committee

The court itself is a purely administrative device: it does not itself give either punishment or treatment. The Ingleby Committee (see p. 148), which held its first meeting in November 1956, is empowered to inquire into and make recommendations on the working of the law in England and Wales relating to proceedings and the powers of the courts in respect of juveniles brought before the courts as delinquent, or as being in need of care or protection or being beyond control; the constitution, jurisdiction and procedure of juvenile courts; the remand home, approved school, and approved probation home systems; and the prevention of cruelty to and exposure to moral and physical danger of juveniles.

CHAPTER VI

PHYSICIAN AND CHILD

THE SPECIALITY OF GENERAL PRACTICE

It is a commonplace that medicine in general practice differs markedly from hospital medicine. In hospital, to quote Dr Rickman again, 'the patient is drawn into a region where he is isolated from usual social contacts and interests, and is examined by a number of hospital departments which have specialized on one or other aspect of the mechanism of his body or mind'.[1] There comes a time, however, for all but the few, when the child must return to his own environment. The catchment area of a hospital is large, and the homes of the children attending it are necessarily diverse. It is at a severe disadvantage in obtaining information about the patient as a child in his home. The visiting staff of social workers from the hospital give valuable help, but as they are investigating over the whole of the hospital's catchment area, they can but rarely know a child or a family over a period of years, and their knowledge cannot be deep.

Someone has to take the high technicalities of the hospital and relate them to the peculiarities of the child's environment. From the nature of things the hospital consultant cannot do this, and the social worker is not equipped to do it. The only person who is properly placed and intellectually equipped to perform this special task is the general practitioner. To do so he needs to turn the same interested eye towards the workings and failures of social life as to the workings and failures of the body. R. J. H. F. Pinsent wrote:

Very many of the problems of childhood with which the general practitioner will be confronted are non-clinical in that they do not concern disease as he has been taught to regard it. Many such problems arise from the child's adjustment to the social environment of its home,

[1] J. Rickman, *B.M.J.* **2** (1947), 363.

its parent or its school. The nervous child, the fractious child, the child whose school progress is slow, the bed-wetter, or even the perfectly normal child, may be brought up to visit the doctor when a family situation has got beyond control.... Once parents have seen the full ritual of examination applied to their child they will more readily accept a diagnosis and prognosis in which they themselves are involved.[1]

THE CHILD IN TROUBLE

The delinquent child has committed some offence against society: has stolen, for example, and been discovered. Not all children who steal are discovered and not all those who are discovered are charged and find their way to the juvenile court. It is obviously useful and meaningful, from the administrative point of view, to label the child who is convicted of theft at the juvenile court as a delinquent and the child who is referred to the doctor by his parents because he 'takes things' as neurotic, maladjusted or disturbed. The investigator might well conclude, however, that there were many factors in common in the two children and that they could usefully be regarded together as children in trouble.

Children may be troublesome to others or troubled in themselves. When either sort of child is referred to the doctor, he is bound, as part of the ordinary doctor-patient relationship, to review the circumstances which have led to the child's being in trouble and to consider how best, in his judgment, he can assist him to find a place in his environment. This will involve consideration of the unique child, his endowment and his home circumstances, including the temperament and character of his parents and sibs, together with the way of life of the neighbourhood where the family has its home.

'Good' children

It is clear that the child who is troublesome to other people is much more likely to be presented to the doctor than the child whose difficulties are—anyhow as yet—only his own. The physically or mentally handicapped child, the child who offends against

[1] *An Approach to General Practice* (London, 1953), pp. 108–9.

85

the folkways, mores, laws, or ethical standards; the child who is noisy, truculent, rude, destructive, demanding and unruly, is the child about whom action is taken.

Teachers tend to be preoccupied by the behaviour of the turbulent child, as indeed are parents and neighbours. Distracting in the classroom, unruly in the playground, when punishment fails he is much more likely to be referred for investigation than a quiet and troubled child. Maladjustment does not always show itself in aggressive or troublesome conduct; indeed, quiet and passive behaviour may overlay deep emotional disturbance.[1]

The quiet worried nail-biter, the withdrawn and docile deaf child, may easily be overlooked in the press of everyday life in the classroom. Any unusual attribute in the child might be of relevance (and many attributes which receive the high approval of teachers, parents and those in charge of children's homes should be noted) in finding a troubled child.

Children are rarely 'as good as gold', 'always neat and tidy', 'always wanting to stay in', 'never wanting to mix with other children', and if they are, taking into account current norms and their local variation, then such children are, if no more than statistically, abnormal. Some may feel that all children have an undeniable right to a certain amount of happiness. Undoubtedly a great deal of educational and mental hygiene practice is based upon that view, which has so grown in importance over the past half century that, for example, the opening words of the White Paper which preceded the 1944 Act were: 'The Government's purpose in putting forward the reforms described in this Paper is to secure for children a happier childhood....'[2]

This is an attitude to life, however, which does not draw unanimous approval even within the British Isles, and no one has the right to enforce it upon children whose parents or guardians may think otherwise. This may present itself as a problem from time to time, particularly in children's homes run by religious organisations or in families where the parents have an attitude to life which is

[1] *Report of the Committee on Maladjusted Children* (H.M.S.O. 1955), p. 23.
[2] *Educational Reconstruction* (H.M.S.O. 1943), p. 1.

rigid and severe or where they conform to some minority code. The inescapable fact is that, just as couples marry for better or for worse, so children have their parents for better or for worse. Because he is not himself a Christian Scientist or a spiritualist, vegetarian, anthroposophist, anarchist or communist, that does not give the educationist or doctor the right to abolish the sect, prohibit the reproduction of the members and prevent them from bringing up their children to their own way of life. That their children are different and their behaviour not as other children's is not surprising. The child may well get into difficulties or manifest signs of stress at school principally because, it may be thought, he 'isn't like other children' and is called upon to carry too heavy a burden. But he cannot be taken into care (see p. 138) merely because his parents subscribe to a different way of life. An individual judgment has to be made for each child. Can this child cope, or be helped to cope, with life as he finds it? Where the answer is 'no', there are two very difficult alternatives: to change the parents' attitude to life or to prove, in law, that the child is neglected, cruelly treated or otherwise deprived. Success in either course may open up a whole array of problems and may prove only doubtfully beneficial to the child. It is wilful neglect, in law, to deny 'proper' medical attention on grounds of religious objection. Prosecution is only likely to occur if a child dies, when the parents may be accused of manslaughter. Parents may bring an action for assault against a doctor who treats a child against their wishes. Where the alternative, say to a blood-transfusion, is death, the action is not likely to be successful.[1]

Gifted children

Exceptionally gifted children may come from widely differing homes. 'Born musicians' may be born into families quick to recognise their talents. A young Yehudi in a Menuhin family sets the family doctor a pretty problem from time to time.[2] The boy is abnormal; the education and training his eager parents want to give him is contrary to accepted principles. The question for the

[1] J. S. Tapsfield, *B.M.J.* I (1958), 1298.
[2] R. Magidoff, *Yehudi Menuhin* (London, 1956).

doctor is: Is this child, within this family, fit to submit to this training? The law forbids the training of a child under twelve years of age to take part in performances of a dangerous character, his exploitation in begging or his presence in the bar of licensed premises; it forbids a child's being taken into houses of ill-repute or a girl's being trained in the ways of prostitutes. Otherwise—providing it is not 'employment' (see p. 167) and the child is receiving efficient education (see p. 165)—the parents are free to bring up their child as they please. These restrictions are far removed from the problem which the outstandingly gifted child may present to the doctor. Few of the great men and women of these islands had 'normal' childhoods; yet all, for the past century, have been more or less in the care of a general practitioner. He has seen, too, exceptional children whose abilities have been despised, warped or neglected, who have been pampered or over-driven. There is little that he can do by interference; there is a great deal he can accomplish, however, if he has taken care to see that as the family doctor he has established an adequate relationship with the parents, by orientating the parents' thoughts to the problem which he anticipates. Action rests with the parents, and it may not be until there is factual confirmation of the doctor's prognosis that the parents are ready to listen to and perhaps act upon his advice. But if he has early set out to win the confidence of the parents, advice may well be proffered and accepted at the earliest opportunity.

PITFALLS IN GENERAL PRACTICE

In practice there are difficulties. The family doctor must not only accumulate knowledge about his neighbourhood, but teach himself to order that information and to move among it in a workmanlike way, so that he may feel professionally competent. Furthermore, he needs to develop the ability not only to understand the observable facts about his neighbourhood, but also to approach in a careful, workmanlike and professional manner, the subjective components of local life. He must learn to be at home with feelings, with loving and hating, being frightened, angry and bored, having ideas and ideals. He must learn to proceed slowly and carefully among these feelings. Rudolf Virchow wrote more than a century ago in his *Die Medizinische Reform*: 'The physicians are the natural attorneys of the poor, and social problems fall to a large extent within their jurisdiction.'[1]

Today we understand that social life presents its problems to rich and poor, old and young. Here is an example of one such problem:

Sandra, aged three plus, is the daughter of a commercial traveller for a bicycle firm, a man of nearly forty who had met his wife—the daughter of a customer—on his rounds in inner working-class London. She is some ten years younger than he. They live, now, in a small house on a housing estate. They married when they discovered the girl was pregnant. The husband is often away at night and the wife says she is lonely on the new estate and frightened at night. She took Sandra to the doctor, with vague complaints to the effect that Sandra 'wasn't very well'.

On examination, the child appeared pale and underweight. She stood with her head down, biting her lower lip. She held her mother's hand tightly with her left hand and clasped a rather grubby teddy with her right arm. Physical examination showed no abnormality.

Conversation with the mother elicited that she had been married before, at eighteen, to a National Service man who had been killed a few months after the marriage. She had never been fond of her second husband. They had met at drinking parties at the hotel where he stayed on his rounds. If they had a common interest it was alcohol—and, then, as a result, her pregnancy. They both drink a great deal still, which leaves them short of money; they are suspicious of each other, both as to money and physical fidelity and both are violent when they quarrel.

The mother recounted that their last quarrel was about a week ago. On that occasion she was upstairs bathing Sandra, preparatory to putting her to bed. She had been worrying about how to find the money to pay the rent next day, for they were already in arrears. Her husband, who had been drinking, came in and stumbled over the pram in the dark. The wife left Sandra in the bath, and switched on the passage light, and the husband threw at her a tin of peas which he saw lying with other shopping in the pram. The wife, in a towering rage, threw it back, put on her hat and coat and went to her sister, some

---

[1] Quoted in H. E. Sigarist, *Medicine and Human Welfare* (Yale Univ. Press, 1941), p. 93.

eight miles away—leaving Sandra in the bath alone with an angry and far from sober father. The quarrel did not appear to be remarkably different from those of the past eighteen months or so.

Common sense

Sandra was the doctor's patient. She was being reared, it might be judged, in a home where nothing could flower. The problem, clearly, was not only hers: both the parents were in a painful muddle. In such a case there is a temptation to reach for a universal hack-saw, to say the marriage is hopeless—the sooner it is broken up the better. Why make heavy weather of the thing? Common sense tells one the marriage must end.

Common sense is a very valuable thing. It teaches, among other things, that for the surgeon the hack-saw, or indeed any tool, is not of universal application. The fact is that the couple are both Irish and Catholic. Short answers of common sense—'It was good enough for me, it is good enough for you', 'It's because mothers go out to work', 'Drink is always the trouble'—sound as disgracefully stupid in the consulting room as 'Always carry an old potato', 'I don't catch cold, why should you?', or 'It's because they eat cooked food'.

Avoidance

The problem might be avoided: the doctor might say, 'There is nothing wrong with Sandra.' In fact there is a great deal wrong with Sandra, and with her parents—and mother knows it—knows enough anyhow, so far as her daughter is concerned, to bring her to the doctor for advice. Problems of this sort can be avoided for really quite a time.

Caroline was eleven plus, the illegitimate daughter of the youngest and single daughter of a small farmer in a remote corner of eastern England. Caroline's mother kept house and was completely dominated by her mother. Caroline rarely went out of doors; she could sometimes be seen peering out of the farm upstairs windows. She was always dressed in a velvet frock with a lace collar. In six years Caroline had made less than thirty attendances at school. Whenever the education authority caught up with the child's absences, the private doctor was summoned smartly and he issued a certificate—'asthma'.

Donald Ford reports a child of twelve whose problem was avoided within the administrative county of London.

> I remember...a child who came from a home where his mother had continually treated him as a baby and refused to recognise that her son was growing up. In the end the mother was removed to a mental institution a very sick woman and the plight of her son was brought to light; he was taken into care immediately.
> The boy was twelve years old when he came into care; he had never been taught to care for himself in any way at all and was only with difficulty persuaded to stand upright and walk. He had to be trained to use the W.C. as would a child of eighteen months of age. He could neither dress nor undress himself. He could scarcely hold a spoon in his hands. All through his life he will suffer from a permanent curvature of the spine because he was scarcely, if ever, allowed to adopt an erect position by his mother.[1]

'In the end'...'immediately'! The problems of both children could not fail to be observed; yet for years it would seem, they were avoided and the child, probably in both cases, irreparably damaged.

Reassurance and exaggeration

Somewhere between the common-sense short answer and avoidance lies too facile reassurance: 'She will be all right', 'She will grow out of it'. Maybe she will, but the mother is sufficiently concerned about her child to consult the doctor. Reassurance, like common sense, has its place. It *may* be all that is required. On the other hand, nothing can contribute more effectively to a parent's feeling of inadequacy than cheerful but unacceptable reassurance. Professor Illingworth writes:

> Some practitioners and paediatricians evince little interest in behaviour problems and fail to give the parents the advice which they need....All too often the mother is merely told that 'It's his nerves', 'It is just naughtiness', 'He just wants a good smacking', 'He is just spoilt', 'He will grow out of it'—all statements which give the mother no help at all.[2]

---

[1] D. Ford, *The Deprived Child* (London, 1955), p. 21.
[2] R. S. Illingworth, *The Normal Child* (London, 1953), p. 216.

He warns, too, that:

All normal children have behaviour problems. It is wrong to think that children with these problems are in any way abnormal, naughty, nervous or maladjusted. Many of the problems are merely part and parcel of the normal development of the child. Wisely managed they are short-lived. Improperly managed they may become exaggerated, last for years and become moulded into the character which a man will carry with him for the rest of his life.

Just as the organism and environment are inseparable, interactive and interdependent, so too are the social, emotional, mental and physical aspects of life. The physical examination itself is concerned with both genetic and environmental factors, inextricably inter-playing: the question is how far in either direction it is useful to pursue orderly inquiry—how far, for example, the individual investigator is equipped to follow the interplay of love and hate within a family.

Projection

Love and hate cannot be found in a bottle any more than can sexual desire. Demonstrably necessary components of all three may be up there on the shelf; but loving, hating and desiring are something a person feels: they are subjective experiences. The mistake is to assume that what the observer feels, the other person must.

Mrs Andrews, though only twenty-three, weighed nearly eighteen stone. Her son, six weeks old, was in the pram. The equipment was shiny and new. Mrs Andrews had been shopping. She noticed that the infant had slipped down to the point of disappearing under the clothes. She stopped the pram, moved to the side and said, 'Come on, you are getting lazy.'

Now some, of course, recognise what they call 'lazy babies'; but before anyone would accept the judgment of this mother, independent and supporting evidence would be necessary, for it might be suspected that it was upon the mother that flesh was hanging heavily and that she was projecting her own feelings upon the infant son. It is stupid, if not dangerous, merely to project one's own thoughts and feelings upon another, if one wishes to understand him. A quiet and cultivated acquaintance with one's own thoughts and feelings is required. Clearly our individual ability to do this varies and so too does our own individual experience of life. To be married and with a family may help a man to understand family problems. It does not follow, though, that all married people understand family problems or that those who are single cannot understand the thoughts and feelings of the married.

Sympathy and empathy

It is sometimes said that sympathy is necessary in order to understand another's thoughts and feelings. Sympathy, however, does not of itself give insight.

Father was sitting in his study looking at rather than reading the evening paper. He had played golf in the afternoon, he had been working very late the night before. He was hungry for his dinner—and he had to go out afterwards. He felt drearily discontented and sleepy. He heard the quick feet of his small daughter Letty. She flung the door open. Father sat up, put the paper aside and opened his arms and legs. Letty was in a rage. She flung herself at father's waistcoat. He closed his arms and legs about her and bent his face to the top of her head. It was some time before the first sob came and much longer before he spoke: 'You poor old thing. Take it easy: take it easy.' He smiled above the child's head, waiting for Laetitia to recover.

The father's feelings were in sympathy with his daughter: his feelings were changed by her entry, he felt with her; but his subjective experience was quite different from the anger of his daughter and her need for his steady comfort. In human life, in everyday affairs, the father's feelings were exactly what the situation demanded. He and his daughter were sympathetic just as the instruments of the orchestra may be symphonic. The father's feelings do not necessarily give him insight to his daughter's feelings: he may be the best father in the world and be incapable of conceiving the rage of a three-year-old against her five-year-old brother. Family life, in practice, may make only small demands upon our ability to feel into other people—to empathise.

In everyday life we feel into the cinema screen and laugh at shadows and cry—and feel a bit foolish about the tears when the lights go up. We feel into the play at the theatre, we 'catch the spirit' of a party or a meeting: we are 'taken out of ourselves'. Perhaps the audience at a boxing show as the bout becomes 'exciting' may be divided into those who give and those who receive the blows. We can learn quietly and gently to avoid the dangers of projection and to explore the possibility of empathisation, to cultivate our innate ability to feel other people's lives.

Limits

There are natural limits to the exploration. In each one of us, because we are all the persons we are, there are mental states and human actions which disgust us, which 'we cannot understand'. It is as well to recognise this. For one, drunkenness may be utterly disgusting, or it may be theft or homosexuality or heterosexual perversion. These limits are not absolutely fixed any more than the revulsion to blood and the knife is necessarily permanent: they exist, however, and must be recognised. This recognition is an important aid to a doctor's confidence in moving about among his own thoughts and feelings. All these things have to be accomplished by dint of his own effort. Occasionally a few have the assistance of others pursuing the same goal; yet even so the going is by no means easy, as the following quotation concerning an experience at the Tavistock Clinic will show:

A group of eight doctors met weekly to discuss our own cases, as a research seminar. We were a varied group, with only one thing in common—that we were all doctors in general practice. The sexes, ages, and nationalities were mixed. We had the usual tensions of any therapeutic group, for that is what we inevitably became (in a mild sort of way). We got to know each other really well and we recognised each other's patterns, idiosyncrasies, and weaknesses, and were fully conscious that everyone else was just as aware of our own deficiencies.

We gradually became more and more cognizant of the intricacies of the hackneyed doctor-patient relationship, and the traditional 'bottle' was given a little extra meaning. Listening to our colleagues relating their own cases (with some cunning and judicious guidance from the psychiatrist leader), it soon became apparent how varied and different we all were in our individual approaches to the patient, and how we all expected him to conform to certain patterns of behaviour, each of us taking it for granted that our own brand of expectation was the correct one.

Most of us learned to examine our own attitudes in the light of these discoveries, and our increasing ability to acknowledge and accept criticism was a very noticeable by-product. Incidentally, we became highly critical of each other—not much was missed by us, and indeed we were often brutal. This was where the psychiatrist was called upon to exercise all his skill in keeping the temperature at a reasonable level. We began to understand what he meant when he spoke about the 'apostolic function' of the doctor—one of his pet hobby-horses. We were also given the opportunity of discussing difficulties concerning our own cases with one of the psychiatrists at the Tavistock Clinic (other than the seminar leader).

All this helped to increase our elasticity, so necessary in dealing with patients in general practice, reducing tension, and, most important, removing some of our own guilt feelings towards patients. We also noted that the patient responded favourably to our new type of approach and our new style of listening. We got to know something about what could be done for different patients, who could benefit by psychotherapy, and who should not be referred to a psychiatrist.

We even attempted psychotherapy ourselves. At first we looked for startling and dramatic cases, and in fact got what appeared to be amazing results—so much so that it made some of us over-ambitious. But after a bit we learned that beginners' luck did not continue to hold, and with some miserable failures we gradually dropped attempts at major psychotherapy and became more aware of our own limitations and more sensitive to what we could and should attempt, finally settling down to a type of therapy varying with our own individual skill and inclination. In my own case a combination of ventilation, reassurance, and counselling.

My personal development in the group was one of wonder at what was attempted and achieved by certain other members of the group, and then came a remarkable result in one of my early cases, a bit of magic which rather over-stimulated me. I was soon disillusioned by a dismal failure, and finally settled to my present level of treatment.[1]

TREATMENT

In the chapters which follow concerning the exceptional home, the infant at home, the child at school, and the handicapped child, the facilities for maintaining child health and the means available for

[1] P. R. Saville, *B.M.J.* I (1957), 158.

the management and sometimes prevention of difficulties are mentioned in some detail. The amount of description of explicit therapeutic measures is small. The reasons are, first, that where detailed therapeutic processes exist, they are applicable, for the most part by the specialist of clinic or hospital. Secondly, the early detection, prevention, and management of disease where there is a recognised large environmental factor (other than in the public health sense) are not well understood. The facilities which are available have developed empirically and their application is likewise empirical. Thirdly, physical treatment will be symptomatic or inappropriate if the causes of ill-health are attributable to environmental factors.

Some changes can be made to the environment; but particularly for a child these are relatively restricted. What can conveniently be called the Public Health control of environment is understood, generally accepted and largely enforceable. Only a few environmental changes concerning the education, care and protection of a child are understood, generally accepted and enforceable.

Therapeutic relationship

The child who is troubled or in trouble needs help not so much with the objective aspects but with the subjective components of his culture. The first therapeutic step in these matters is the establishment of the doctor–patient relationship: the therapeutic relationship. The object is to orientate the patient to where his difficulty is judged to lie, and to assist him to find a solution acceptable to himself and his culture.

Sometimes there is no solution. The adult male homosexual provides an example. X had been a patient for some years. He had had every possible treatment without any success, and the time had come for the doctor to say that nothing could be done for him. He was not promiscuous, did not seek out little boys and fought against his feelings. He had formed a happy, stable and exclusive relationship in which there was a physical component with a passive, rather younger man. The patient made great efforts to break the attachment. The physician knew that his statement: 'Nothing can be done' would be countered by a very real and urgent question, in spite of its seeming illogicality: 'What am I to do?' What advice could the physician give in such a case? Suppose that the physician had himself no overriding objection to homosexuality; nevertheless he could not ignore the fact that two consenting males who perform in private a homosexual act commit a criminal offence. That fact he could not ignore, even if he could also recall satisfactory and stable households where two women live similarly together; even if he remembered that the patient's problem would disappear in France—or in Britain, if the law were changed. The law has not been changed, and the doctor must in the interests of his patient accept the morals of the society within which the patient lives, even if they do not happen to be his own. There is no solution, but the patient will require comfort and support from his physician: his health will depend upon this relationship.

A patient like Sandra (see p. 89) may present the doctor with problems for which there is but a partial solution. The most hopeful feature in this case is that her mother has sought advice. The immediate goal is for the mother to come to see that Sandra's condition is symptomatic of the family situation. Sandra may well need physical treatment to remedy the damage of distress and to enable her to withstand it more efficiently. Similarly mother and father may be in physical need and the offer of physical treatment may well provide the opportunity to direct the parents' attention towards the basic difficulty. Environmental changes may be considered. The family might do better in the mother's own neighbourhood if it can there be in effective relationship with the extended family, thus providing Sandra with aunts, uncles, cousins and grandparents with whom she may realise an effective tie. Mother may well be more 'at home' with better family contacts, her life may become less lonely and better integrated. The relationship between husband and wife might become less intense if it were lived out in the wider context, rather than contained within the restricted house on a new estate, where the social contacts are minimal, and if they are made, essentially 'exploratory' rather than imposed by blood relationship. Furthermore, the pattern of behaviour of the couple might well be within accepted limits in their original neighbourhood. Should there be a concentration of Catholics there the whole family would benefit from that support, and for Sandra attendance at the Catholic school and at church might effect a marked improvement.

Whether the parents will be prepared to face their own difficulties can be discovered only by assay; but the physical assistance and environmental changes alone will only alleviate their condition. Perhaps the couple will accept reference to the Catholic Marriage Advisory Council. Such acceptance is largely dependent upon the doctor's ability to make the parents feel that he is concerned for them: that he has entered into a therapeutic relationship with them.

Sandra's symptoms may clear up; but she may be deeply disturbed and in need not only of the understanding friendship of her doctor, but also of the services of the child guidance clinic.

Sometimes the doctor, with his knowledge of prognosis, is the only person who sees clearly the steps that can be taken to minimise the effect of illness on the life of a family.

Mrs Winter comes to see the doctor, who is new to the district. She is the wife of a poor smallholder, whose home is a scattered hamlet in the west country; the nearest town is fifteen miles away. The couple are in their mid-twenties; there is an infant daughter, and a son Brian, now nearly five. When Brian was an infant, the mother reported, he gave his parents much concern. He looked like a little old man rather than a baby, and she noticed his skin was rough and yellow; he was a 'lazy baby'; he would not take his food readily. His tongue seemed large for his mouth.

Brian was taken to hospital, where according to his mother, she was instructed to give tablets regularly to him. She took him back from time to time for supervision and was always told to continue with the tablets regularly. She probably never sought any explanation of the infant's condition: she was certainly never given any which she could remember.

Brian is now nearly old enough to go to school. He is a large boy, difficult to control, and with a voracious appetite. At nearly five, he has no words and is not house-trained. His mother finds Brian 'naughty', 'a handful'. 'I can't do anything with him. He gets on my nerves. He upsets my husband. I don't like leaving him with the baby.'

It is not until Brian is nearly school age that the couple decide to 'speak to the doctor'. They are informed that the child is defective. Mrs Winter, although prepared to recount her difficulties with Brian resents the diagnosis of mental defect and angrily rejects it.

The doctor has been presented with a permanent feature of his practice: Brian, who is mentally defective. He is also presented with the necessity of leading the whole family towards the understanding that it, too, is in possession of an as yet unrecognised permanent feature. His object must be the optimum health of the whole family. He must see that the right questions are asked by the members of the family at the right time. Of the objective environmental questions which he must consider, the following may be selected as examples: There are four members of the family—what is to be done? Private homes are beyond the means of a poor smallholder: there are long waiting lists for publicly provided accommodation. Children do better, by and large, at home, and parents are often reluctant to part with their children except when they are quite unmanageable. The family lives in a rural area and there is no occupation centre available. In the child's interest the family ought to consider moving to a large town, where training would be available for the child. If they consider moving, can they get a house? Can the father get a job in a town when the only skill he knows is one which provides a living in the country? Anyhow, you cannot leave a smallholding by giving a week's notice. What if the wife and husband are bound to live in the country for the sake of their health? If the child remains in the present home, what will happen then? On the subjective questions, an assessment of all the members' feelings, of shame, anger, anxiety, fear, has to be made. The happiness, social efficiency and physical health of all the members of the family, including Brian, may depend upon the doctor's ability to relate the diagnosis to the peculiarities of the child's environment.

Sometimes the doctor may effectively limit damage and witness what is truly cure, if he is alerted to watch for it. It occurs perhaps many times a day, when he assures a mother that the appearance of the infant's mouth is normal, that little boys often have erections, that the child is not 'going bad inside' because he has missed a stool or two.

A cool and matter-of-fact approach aimed at reducing adult tensions is of importance in handling sexual irregularities in children, and made early enough may do much to prevent harmful results to the child. A child who has had some sexual experience is likely to be in difficulties for two main reasons.

First, he may experience pain and fear. He may be physically hurt, damaged, and overwhelmed. The child's problem is then a twofold one of actual physical damage and the associated fear. He is comparable to a child who has been cruelly beaten, has had a road accident or has been attacked by an incapacitating disease.

Secondly, the child may suffer no physical damage; the episode may have been essentially exploratory or pleasure-seeking, or both. The child may well know that the activity is forbidden, and in consequence may suffer guilt. Few parents give their children explicit sexual instruction together with explicit rules and prohibitions, so that the child may know with some accuracy what is permitted and what forbidden as he does, for example, concerning possessions, and what is and what is not stealing. Parents avoid explicit training, and rely on passive learning, precisely because of their anxiety to rear their children 'correctly'.

The difficulties of the conscientious parent are considerable. The whole subject is emotionally highly charged, the parents themselves implicated, and not always certain of their own successful adaptation to the mores. There are conflicting views about sexual conduct, and varieties of ways advocated for training and informing children. Among them the main element of agreement—because of the high emotional charge—is the profound and far-reaching importance of 'proper' teaching. For these reasons, parents rely sometimes on arbitrarily stated prohibitions, often quite contrary in tone to the rest of their methods with their children, and sometimes upon passive learning. In fact, a great deal of social learning and adaptation takes place passively, without specific cortical activity. Children adapt themselves to the required norms. Now sexual activity is by no means exclusively presented as 'wrong' or as limited to marriage. Conversation, jokes, advertisements, literature, drama, radio and television, present sex quite otherwise. There is no reason to suppose that the child does not make both explicit and implicit adaptations to these presentations.

Two inferences appear to be possible: few, if any, normal children can grow up in Britain without acquiring some notion that sexual behaviour is endowed with penalties and pleasures quite different from those, say, associated with eating; and on the other hand, few children grow up today with quite explicit standards of right or wrong. Accordingly, few children will feel no guilt when they are found to be masturbating, exploring each other, or attempting connection either with other children or adults. Their feelings will be quite different, for example, from those of little boys who in the company of adults or other children pass their water in the gutter in the high street, or suck an ice-cream while walking along. There will always be some feeling of 'wrong', even if it is no stronger than that of little boys who are discovered by an adult 'seeing who can pee the furthest' or sucking ice-cream they have failed to pay for. But few children are likely to have a strong feeling of guilt; most are more likely to be perplexed and confused and to respond quickly to a matter-of-fact and reasonably coherent explanation.

The attitude of society may be part cause of the difficulties. Any act of a child, whether physically painful, indifferent, or pleasurable, guilt-laden or free, which provokes intense anxiety and activity among his circle of adults, may induce fear and do extensive damage to the child. The whole of the child's world may collapse.

Sylvia, aged nine, lived in a dock area. Her father was a seaman and her mother worked all day as a waitress. She was a rather lonely little girl, used to the company of adults. She spent a lot of time in the lodging-house next door and the wife there gave her meals and kept an eye on her. One of the men lodgers she called 'uncle'. She was fond of him and enjoyed his company. He fondled her, and there was ultimately a sexual connection. She found the relationship warm, loving and intimate. There was, of course, one man she loved above all others and to this man, her father, she offered when he came home a relationship which was warm, loving and intimate. He rejected her advances. Father thrashed Sylvia, beat his wife, fought 'uncle'. There was a criminal charge and Sylvia was sent for treatment.

Sylvia could not have been a more innocent little girl. Because of her innocence, her world collapsed around her. Her parents were a sensible couple, but they were overwhelmed by shame, fear, and anger. Sylvia's behaviour was unacceptable. Her environmental experience had taken her beyond the mere words of thousands of growing children: 'I want to marry you, Daddy, when I grow up.' 'I think it is silly that you can't marry your brother. You've got Daddy, Mummy, why can't I have Bobby?' 'They *are* the nicest people in the world, aren't they?' This having occurred, disaster came to her—and by way of her father. Her first need was for the general reduction of the emotional tension of those around her, then some coherent explanation of the situation and then a healing relationship with the child psychiatrist that would endure until she was able to reconstruct her life again.

Guidance

The methods of investigation and treatment for the troublesome and troubled child, whether he is referred by parents, school, local authority or juvenile court to private doctor, hospital or clinic, derive from the teachings of child psychology and are usually furnished by the child guidance clinics. The clinics are unevenly distributed throughout the country and there is a lack of trained personnel. There is in consequence often considerable delay in obtaining treatment. The development of special classes for maladjusted children within schools has taken place in London, Oxford, and elsewhere; these provide satisfactorily for some children in trouble at school and help to relieve some of the pressure on the clinics.[1] The clinics vary in structure, provision and methods, but they all approximate more or less to the following form.

[1] V. L. Kahan and J. R. Fish, *Med. Off.* **95** (1956), 149.

Investigation

The child is investigated in three main ways: physically, psycho-logically and socially. He is seen by the psychiatrist, who examines him and assesses his psychiatric state. The psychologist investigates the child's mental abilities and what he has done with them—that is, his educational attainments. From her observation of the child in the standard situation of the tests and, more directly, by means of tests designed for the purpose, she also assesses the child's emotional state. The psychiatric social worker investigates the milieu, so that she can understand the child within his family and the family within its neighbourhood. The three investigations are integrated for the purposes of a diagnosis and for the planning of treatment.

Treatment

Arrangements may be made elsewhere for the treatment of physical defects.

If the child has some educational difficulty remedial teaching may be suggested. The fact that a boy cannot make head or tail of, say, arithmetic, may be an important factor in his unacceptable conduct. The cause may range all the way from the rare brain lesion to the simple fact that he was away with a cold when a key lesson was given. Children may well manufacture an arithmetic of their own; if so, it has to be unravelled and then reknitted up as quickly and neatly as possible. There may be difficulties at school to be adjusted: the child may be in the wrong 'stream': he might manage better if in one stream for one subject and another for another.

Most child guidance clinics either employ or refer cases to a speech-therapist. There has been since the time of the work among difficult evacuated children during the war a great increase of interest in speech difficulties and a corresponding advance in skill in dealing with some of the defects and underlying causes.

The psychiatric social worker has her contribution to make in the therapeutic phase: she cannot alter the environment, she is equipped with no axe or hack-saw, but she can win the confidence of the family, helping them to gain insight into their problems, inter-preting what is happening in the clinic to the family and what is happening in the family to the clinic.

Play-therapy

When emotional difficulties are involved, the psychiatrist may conduct a series of interviews with one or both parents. For the child play-therapy is frequently provided if he has no fundamental, emotional or temperamental limitations. The object is to explore the content of his mental life, and the method is based upon the 'therapeutic' relationship—an understanding of the patient that can be achieved by a partial participation of the therapist in the problems involved. It is usual to refer to the therapy as either intensive or supportive. In the first, the object is to effect person-ality changes by uncovering the relatively deep-rooted bases of the child's difficulties. The second has the object of buttressing the patient's existing defences and is used either where he is regarded as unsuitable for the intensive type because of the nature of his illness and his poor adjustment, or where he is himself psycho-logically stable, but the unsatisfactory situation in which he finds himself is unalterable. A physically handicapped child, for example, might fall into either category. A few children are so disturbed that only mental hospital treatment is suitable; but the adult ward of a mental hospital is no place for a child.[1] Some special provision is now available. The seeking of help is of itself regarded as an important factor in psychotherapy. Unlike the adult, who ordinarily seeks psychological treatment himself, the child finds his way to it at the bidding of others. The likelihood that the child will continue to attend is greater if his parents are the ones to seek help. But for a good relationship—rapport—to be established he must also find some satisfaction in the sessions.

[1] The Royal Medico-Psychological Association in its Memorandum *In-Patient Accommodation for Child and Psychiatric Patients* (July 1957) recommends, *inter alia*, that in-patients' wards—not less than twenty beds per population of half-a-million—should be provided for children in association with local child psychiatric or child guidance clinics. It is also recommended that in each regional hospital board area there should be a unit of not less than twenty-five beds for a residual group needing prolonged care.

The play room provides opportunities for diagnosis as well as for therapy. The role of the play-therapist is mainly passive and the design of the room and its equipment is such that a wide range of activity is possible for the child. By observation of what he does (or does not do) of his expression, posture and movements, and by attention to his conversation, a judgment of his difficulties may be made. It is sometimes found that early play, which schematically may be regarded as belonging to the diagnostic phase, is itself therapeutic: the child is less of a nuisance, less inhibited, relieved, as though he were in part purged—or, as some say, there has been catharsis.

The object of play-therapy, as with adult psychotherapy, is not alone to purge the child, but to give him some understanding of his own difficulties. The child proceeds at his own pace, but with the assistance of the play-therapist. A little girl who is in conflict with her brother may play regularly with a doll in the play room and regularly and unmistakably be aggressive, perhaps brutal, to it. The explanation may be obvious to the clinic staff. While this play continues it may be reported that relationships at home have improved. The therapist will help the child to interpret her play so that her emotional attitudes are modified. Thus, success comes when it is plain that the patient realises that she is not angry with the doll and that she has found a solution for her difficulties other than storing up or letting loose her anger. Children may play alone or in groups: group-therapy is usually more helpful when the patient's problems are concerned with getting along with other people.

Such work with children is delicate and skilled, and calls for much ability and knowledge. It rests upon a variety of theoretical foundations deriving from the several deep psychologies or a combination of them. Nevertheless, it is fair to say that it takes the commonplaces of everyday family life—what Tommy did in the park today; what Jane said to the butcher; what Frank drew in his sand tray—and with rare skill directs them to a therapeutic goal.

Child guidance service

Nevertheless, a Committee on Juvenile Delinquency set up by the L.C.C. in its (unpublished) report appears to regard these clinics as inadequate in most particulars.[1] In the report of the Committee on Maladjusted Children, however, it is recommended that there should be a comprehensive child welfare guidance service available for the area of every local education authority, involving a school psychological service, the school health service, and child guidance clinics, 'all of which should work in close co-operation'. More than two hundred child guidance clinics in England and Wales are run in connection with the local education authorities as well as similar provision that may be available through the health service. The report also recommends (among some hundred suggestions) that where children cannot be treated successfully while they remain at home they should for a time go to special classes or boarding establishments. 'The aim should be to provide treatment for parents as well as children, in order to make both the child fit to return home and the home fit to receive him.'

The distribution of the clinics is very uneven. Some areas are reasonably well served.[2] By 1956 the L.C.C., for example, was using twenty-nine hospital and other child guidance clinics and had four centres of its own. In that year there were 516 applications for reference to these four units. The waiting periods were usually two to three months for interview and three to eight months for treatment. In September 1957 a new clinic was opened and another expanded.

[1] *B.M.J.* **2** (1951), 298.
[2] The family doctor will find it convenient to possess the handlist of the National Association of Mental Health (39 Queen Anne St, London, W. 1) which gives the addresses and the names of staff of the recognised child guidance clinics in England and Wales. There is increasing co-operation between the family doctor and the clinics. In Ipswich, for example, over two-thirds of the cases seen at the Department of Child and Family Psychiatry (as it is now called) come direct from general practitioners (*Med. Off.* **99** (1956), 188).

CHAPTER VII

THE EXCEPTIONAL HOME

The physician, concerned with the individual child, seeks to see him in the context of his family and neighbourhood. But that neighbourhood is not self-sufficient. There are economic, political and cultural units dependent upon a much larger context, and with them folkways, mores, laws and ethical principles introduced from the outside.

Many facilities that are available to assist the child and his family are provided by public administration either because the relevant authority is carrying out duties imposed by law, or because it is exercising powers which the law permits. These provisions seek to remedy felt and general needs, and are more or less generally available.

In this chapter some general changes in the constitution of families over the past half-century or so are described, and this is followed by a description of seven types of exceptional homes that may be encountered and the provisions which exist for their help.

Some attempt is made on the one hand to limit the technical administrative detail where it is not the direct concern of the general practitioner, and on the other, to present the description of both facilities and social problems with the doctor in his surgery constantly in mind.

HOUSEHOLDS

In round figures, of the forty-nine million people in Great Britain on the census night in 1951, forty-six and a half millions were found to have occupied thirteen million dwellings and to have formed fourteen and a half million private households, that is, excluding hotels, boarding houses and institutions (which contained two and a half million people). This gives an average number of people per household of rather less than four.

At first sight it would appear that the average household was no bigger than the biological facts would permit: but if each contained a mother, a father, and either one or two children the population would inevitably be falling. In fact the population is rising, and there are a greater number of households smaller, rather than larger, than the average. Indeed, roughly three-quarters of the households produce only one-quarter of the children. There were eight and a quarter million households where there were no children on census night and of these more than one and a half million were single-person households, two-thirds of which consisted of spinsters or widows who were mostly elderly. Now, old ladies can live alone only when they are equipped with the facilities of an industrial culture: electricity, piped water, easily obtained hot water, a host of services (laundry, repair, pre-cooking and preparation, etc.) easily available, and an efficient distribution of goods. The small household can be easily workable only where and so long as there are industrial facilities.

Furthermore in the 1951 census there were nearly two million households that were called 'composite'. They contained eight and a half million persons, of whom 1,240,000 were unattached boarders, but 2,620,000 were persons who formed 980,000 'family nuclei'. Many of the members of these 'family nuclei' would probably have preferred to form households in separate dwellings, for four in every five were married or widowed children or children-in-law of the householder, and well over half of them had children of their own.

The constant reduction in the size of the household has been a characteristic of the past half century and is a major cause of the housing shortage. As the standard of living rises, as the industrial facilities spread, the more nearly is attained most people's felt need of a home—a dwelling that contains the immediate family of the married couple and their dependent children. When children are no longer dependent they tend to set up as a separate household— not yet a home, for that is something for the family.

In the census year there were 120 'habitable' rooms available for every hundred persons. The official standard is 100 rooms per 100 persons and yet twenty per cent of all households were below that minimum. The urgent need for houses—not yet solved in spite of the long post-war building effort; in Birmingham, for example, it is estimated that there are 63,000 families in search of homes[1]—arises from several causes. First, people are attracted to areas where well-paid work is to be found; labour is perforce mobile to some degree, though not always as much as the politician and economist would like. Secondly, the overwhelming majority of houses built between the wars—a period of unprecedented building—were of the three bedroom type with one or two living rooms, and many of these, by the official standard, are under-occupied; even if they were available for division into separate dwellings, they do not easily lend themselves to the process. Thirdly, there are older couples, or sometimes widows, living alone in a larger family house. They regard their house as a stake in the land, as something permanent, as an inheritance. It may be burdensome to maintain; but older people understandably do not want to move and cannot bring themselves to think about a house as something which you buy, like a car, to sell or exchange in a few years or like a room in an hotel which you hire for as long as you want it. Finally, those houses where the rent is restricted by law may sometimes be under-occupied because the rent, fixed on a pre-war basis, is much less than that of the new, smaller flat. One of the purposes of the Rent Act (1957) is to compel movement and a 'better' distribution of room.

Immediate family

The social unit in our society, then, if not the individual, is the married couple and their dependent children—the immediate family. Even this unit is smaller than formerly, for the average completed family of a woman married in 1870 was 5·8 children, whereas that of a woman married in 1925 was 2·2 children.[2] Relatively the difference in family size between the various occupations and social classes has remained little changed during the century. The decline in family size has been characterised more by

[1] *The Times*, 3 August 1956.
[2] D. V. Glass and E. Grebenik (1954), *The Trend and Pattern of Fertility in Great Britain*—a report on the family census of 1946 (Papers of the Royal Commission on Population, vol. VI, H.M.S.O.).

compression of the span of years during which children of a marriage have been born than by widespread spacing. The decline in child-bearing has been greatest in the later stages of married life (within the child-bearing ages) and this decline in fertility with increasing length of married life is especially marked among women of the non-manual occupation groups. The small family pattern is now spreading throughout the whole community and a new stability in family size appears to have been established in recent years.

There has been an undoubted rise in the regard in which children are held and over the half-century a revolution in the standards of child care—a change of very great rapidity in working-class areas from the decades of unemployment to the post-war years—and it is hard for the younger person today to remember that Eleanor Rathbone, the great advocate of family allowances, spoke of the 'disinherited family'. The advent of a wage-earning economy, coupled with the suppression of child labour and the enforcement of compulsory education, had in a very real sense piled up financial difficulties to parenthood. Post-war social services go some way to remedy this; but British social provision pays little attention to the family except when it falls into difficulty or breaks down, and even then tends to afford help in ways which may weaken family ties. This, it is said, is because British social legislation is based on the individual, whereas in France, for example, it is based on the family. The economic burden of children is partly obscured by the general rise in the standard of living and partly relieved by the new provisions; but the burden falls in a period of the life of the parents when their earnings are rarely at a maximum, whereas the share of the nation's income going to those who are no longer responsible for the maintenance of children is increasing and is far greater than it was fifty years ago.[1]

Family limitation

The implication is that somehow the parents succeed in limiting their families, reducing the number of children upon whom they will spend a considerable portion of their income and limiting the

---

[1] R. M. Titmuss, *The Listener*, 15 March 1951, p. 411.

number of child-bearing years. The rise and fall in fertility is unexplained, but it is possible to understand the need people feel to limit their families when they live within a swiftly moving culture and the future is more important than the past—when you are 'too old at forty' and the future is with the children. Whereas in a static society age and wisdom are at a premium, in Britain the parents are subordinated to their children, for whom they desire a higher standard of living than that which they themselves have attained. This desire runs through the whole social structure and the mere arithmetic—unless the increase of material wealth is enormous—necessitates family limitation.

Many peoples besides those in the West practise family limitation. Two common methods—infanticide and abortion—are criminal in Great Britain, and mechanical methods are regarded as sinful by the Catholic Church. Although Colonel Condom was a late seventeenth-century soldier and Annie Besant and Charles Bradlaugh had campaigned for birth control in the nineteenth, it was not until 1930 that the Ministry of Health authorised local authorities to give contraceptive advice to nursing and expectant mothers in whose cases further pregnancy would be detrimental to health. The National Birth Control Council then came into being with the late Lord Horder as president: later it was known as the Family Planning Association and today, with Sir Russell Brain as president, it has 250 clinics in England, Scotland and Wales.[1]

It is not easy to estimate how much contraception is used. There is no legal bar as, for example, in France and Italy, nor, as in those countries today, is there a crusading movement for birth control. The evidence from the Royal Commission[2] must be used with caution, for the sample was small and drawn from two highly-urbanised areas where the numbers of the less well-to-do were disproportionate. Fifty-six per cent of all the women in this sample had used some form of contraception (including abstinence for more than six months, use of the 'safe' period and *coitus*

---

[1] *B.M.J.* I (1957), 1372.
[2] Papers of the Royal Commission (1949) on population, vol. I: *Family Limitation and its Influence on Human Fertility During the Past Fifty Years* (H.M.S.O.).

interruptus). Of those women who had married between 1910 and 1919, forty-one per cent had used some form, and the proportion rose to sixty-seven per cent for women married between 1935–9. There was a greater use in the higher classes and the use of appliances decreased down the social scale.

Among women who had married between 1940 and 1946, fifty-eight per cent in Class I, forty-six per cent in Class II and forty per cent in Class III had planned the number of their children. There was about eight per cent involuntary infertility.

Survival

The increasing certainty of survival is as important a factor in the current attitude to children as is the possibility of controlling their arrival. The expectation of life a century ago for an infant boy was about forty years and for a girl forty-two years. The life table for 1953–5[1] gives 67·46 for infant boys and 72·86 for girls. The reduction in the hazards of birth and of infancy, the enormous improvements in maternity and child welfare and the fair certainty that toddlers will reach maturity enable those who desire a family life responsibly to limit their families. No longer is there the same meaning in the words of the 116th Psalm which the mother repeats in the Church of England Service of Thanksgiving of Women after Child-Birth, commonly called the Churching of Women: 'The snares of death compassed me round about: and the pains of hell gat hold of me', or the alternative 127th Psalm: 'Like as the arrows in the hand of the giant: even so are the young children. Happy is the man that hath his quiver full of them: they shall not be ashamed when they speak with their enemies in the gate.'

The immediate family, the essential unit of our society, is smaller than it has ever been and much more efficient biologically and socially than before; yet its efficiency and very existence is possible only if it has on call a great array of services communally produced. It is possible for two orphans, reared in an institution with no relatives at all, to marry, to obtain a dwelling, to make therein a

[1] *Annual Abstract* (1957) *of Statistics*, no. 94 (H.M.S.O.).

home and have—and become—a family unrecognisable from any other. Few immediate families, of course, are thus dependent only upon their own and communal resources. For most people the family extends beyond the bounds of their household and this 'extended' family still has some social function.

Extended family

The means test—the insistence that the income of all members of a household should be taken into account in assessing need during the period of unemployment—was bitterly resented and was the cause of many single young men and women leaving home. Perhaps as a result there has been a reluctance to investigate the working of the extended family since then. The relationship between the immediate and extended family today has, however, been the subject of at least one study.[1] It is probably true even in the great towns that members—especially wives—of many immediate families are within walking distance of the dwellings of members of their extended family, especially mothers, and that there is regular visiting, continuing verbal communication, mutual assistance and joint observance of family events. The mother-in-law joke is not dead and the tie between a mother and her daughter in working-class areas is still very much alive.

The extended family may be no less real within the middle class but it functions differently. Middle-class men move about in general much more than working-class men, both in their leisure and in pursuit of their occupations, and the salaried worker may often be moved by his employers from place to place. His wife is expected to accompany him and to make him a new home, and both are much more likely to have their home beyond walking distance of members of their extended family. Communication may be frequent and detailed, but written rather than verbal. Services may be regular and valuable: recommendations, introductions and funds transferred by way of the bank. Throughout the class structure the traditional bond of family possessions will hold together the extended family, whether it be a family business in

[1] M. Young and P. Willmott, *Family and Kinship in East London* (London, 1957).

which members work or which they direct, a family profession or real estate. In some rural areas, for example Cumberland, not only may the extended family function together but there may still be a common household on the farm for two or more immediate families, surviving in the traditional joint-family manner.[1] Occasionally, for example among those Jews who are orthodox, there may be strong cultural and religious bonds holding the extended family together for the purpose of traditional observance. At Christmas most families are in touch with their scattered members —except of course many Scots, who defer their celebrations until the New Year.

TYPES OF EXCEPTIONAL HOME

The immediate family establishes itself at marriage and it seeks to make a home within its separate dwelling; there the children of the union grow. Exceptionally, couples experience difficulty or failure in creating their homes; sometimes they are unable or unwilling to maintain them. We must now consider the difficulties of the couple who are without their extended family and therefore heavily dependent upon communal resources; those who are very much dependent upon their extended family, because they cannot secure a separate dwelling; those who secure physically inadequate accommodation in which to make a home; and the unmarried mother and her child. We must consider also those couples who marry, obtain their dwelling and create their home, but do not succeed in having children; they may seek to adopt or foster children. Other families may be endangered by way of quarrels, death or catastrophe. Finally, there is the ineffective couple, who as the result of some defect are cruel to or neglectful of their children, or merely live in squalid incompetence.

The unattached

It is rare for the immediate family to begin without any dependence on the extended family, though it may happen when two sibless orphans or two refugees marry. Again sometimes the marriage is

[1] W. M. Williams, *The Sociology of an English Village* (London, 1956).

disapproved of by both sets of parents and the couple may begin life independently; sometimes one set of parents disapproves. But ordinarily there are some ties either with the older generation or with contemporaries. Family ties need not necessarily mean a physical proximity; many service marriages mean that new families are established perhaps thousands of miles from blood relations; but there is a felt tie between the members of the extended family.

Home nursing and home help

The more remote and the fewer these ties the more likely the couple is to be dependent upon acquaintances and publicly provided assistance in establishing and maintaining the home: to look after the husband while the wife is confined or when she is ill, or to baby-sit.

The local health authority has to provide the necessary service for persons who require nursing in their own homes, either by the direct employment of nurses, or indirectly through the services of voluntary organisations (see p. 160). The local authority may also, with the approval of the Minister of Health, provide domestic help for households where one of the members is an expectant mother, or is ill, lying-in, mentally defective, aged, or a child not over compulsory school age. A charge may be made in suitable cases for this service.

The unattached couple are more likely to need services such as that introduced in Kent, where a child help is provided if there are two or more children and the mother is hospitalised.[1] Not only is it more humane to keep the children at home, to keep the home going, but the cost to the local authority is about half that of institutionalisation. Since 1953 the London County Council has provided a service of child helps to care for two or more children in their own homes when they are temporarily deprived of the care of both parents and there are no other adults in the home at night. The unattached household is a vulnerable unit and it may suddenly find itself in real danger of breaking up.

[1] *Med. Off.* **95** (1956), 91; **97** (1957), 25.

The dependent

When there is no separate accommodation where the couple may create their home, their difficulty may often be that the extended family is much too close and has far too many members. Couples can be found who, though married, continue to live with their own parents for lack of a dwelling. These couples may have married because of the girl's pregnancy. Their difficulty arises from the housing shortage; but it is very similar in nature to that of some couples during the war. While the illegitimate birth-rate doubled during the war, there was a decrease in the extent to which children were conceived out of and born into wedlock.[1] Before the war the parents of seventy per cent of children irregularly conceived had married before the birth of the child. During the war this fell to thirty-seven per cent. The increase in the illegitimacy rate was largely due to enforced separation of parents who would otherwise have married.

Housing

A couple may satisfy their need for a separate dwelling by converting a room or two in the home of one of the parents—usually the girl's. Or they may wait until rooms become available: the landlord fixes the wedding date. The mere fact that the couple marry does not constitute the basis of a claim for housing. Most local authorities evolve a point-system by which statutory over-crowding may be scored and account taken, for example, of tuberculosis among members of the family, length of residence, war service, and so on. Sometimes families are homeless—these are nearly all ineffective families who have been evicted for non-payment of rent or other breach of contract. Eviction is only secured by court order. Provision is made for such families by the local welfare authority, in the former work-house, now referred to as 'short-stay accommodation'.[2]

[1] S. M. Ferguson and H. Fitzgerald, *Studies in the Social Services* (H.M.S.O., 1954).
[2] For an account see Audrey Harvey, 'Operation Pavement', in *New Statesman* (16 March 1957), p. 331.

The inadequately housed

A standard of accommodation is laid down by law for determining when a house is overcrowded; it is designed to secure the proper segregation of the sexes and to restrict the total number of occupants. Local authorities are required to inspect their districts to ascertain the position, and where necessary to provide additional houses. Many premises are still overcrowded, but owing to the lack of alternative accommodation it has been necessary to permit what would otherwise constitute an offence: in each case, however, a licence for the condition has to be obtained.

In England and Wales in 1951 twenty-two per cent of all households were without the exclusive use of a water closet, forty-five per cent without the exclusive use of a fixed bath, and fourteen per cent without the exclusive use of both stove and sink.

Professor Mackintosh summarises the effect of bad housing on children: (a) Bad housing conditions are doubly dangerous in the main infections of childhood; they conduce to early and dangerous attacks and they tend to hinder satisfactory recovery. (b) There is a good deal of evidence that overcrowding as such—the huddling together of human beings in a confined space—may produce adverse effects on health. In practice, however, overcrowding can seldom be separated from other social circumstances; it is one of the manifestations of poverty and is usually accompanied by signs of want.[1] He quotes G. P. Wright and H. P. Wright who, in their study of the influence of social conditions on diphtheria, measles, tuberculosis and whooping cough in early childhood in London, found that while overcrowding was a factor associated with mortality rates in all these conditions, it had an especially strong and close correlation with measles.[2]

It is disappointing after so much effort that the infants born in Newcastle in May and June 1947 who were studied by the late Sir James Spence and his colleagues showed such relatively poor health during their first year, probably in the main because of the

[1] J. M. Mackintosh, *Housing and Family Life* (London, 1952).
[2] *J. Hyg.* (1942), p. 42.

117

poverty of housing.[1] The published report showed that only a fifth of the group escaped illness. The remainder had an average of two illnesses each and some ten per cent had three or more infections. Over four-fifths of the illnesses were infective in origin, the remainder comprising accidents and non-infective skin rashes or illnesses due to congenital abnormalities. Over half of the infective illnesses involved the respiratory system: they ranged from severe 'colds' or tonsillitis to bronchitis and pneumonia. One child in four had a severe cold, one in five had bronchitis, one in twenty-five pneumonia and one in ten whooping cough. Acute digestive upsets accounted for only nine per cent of the illnesses. It was calculated that by the end of the first year of life seven per cent of the children were 'alive but ill'.

But overcrowding and poor housing cannot take the blame for all that goes wrong at home. It has been suggested by D. Hewitt and A. Stewart, after reviewing figures for those areas of England for which acute rheumatism is notifiable, that neither bad housing nor poverty is responsible.[2] They emphasise the greater risk of infection in large families compared with small ones and in children just attaining school-age compared with children of pre-school age. It is suggested that the social incidence of rheumatic fever is the direct result of the social incidence of streptococcal infection. Similarly familial contact rather than numerical crowding or poor housing appears to be the factor of importance in the incidence of tuberculosis.[3] J. W. B. Douglas and J. M. Blomfield, who relied on a sample drawn from all parts of Great Britain and all social classes, found that

overcrowding and generally poor home conditions contributed little to the social group differences in illness. Only lower respiratory infections showed any definite increase, and that a small one, as housing conditions grew worse. The apparent connection between infectious diseases of childhood and poor home conditions was fully explained by the fact that in the worst homes there were more school children

[1] Sir J. C. Spence, W. S. Walton, F. J. W. Miller and S. D. M. Court, *A Thousand Families in Newcastle upon Tyne* (Oxford, 1954), pp. 31–2.
[2] *Brit. J. Soc. Med.* 6, 161.
[3] *B.M.J.* 1 (1957), 633.

to bring infection into the family. Unexpectedly, accidents occurred no more frequently in the worst homes.[1]

Accidents

It is, however, certain that a large proportion of accidents in the home are due to overcrowded and badly-kept houses. The three most important causes of accidents in the home are faulty design and equipment; poor maintenance, particularly of flooring, stair-treads, hand rails, and inadequate lighting; and the human element, ignorance and carelessness.

Today, in the 5–14 age group, violence, taking the form of an accident, is the major cause of death in the male.[2] In the ten years 1940–9 over 60,000 people died from accidents in their homes, compared with 48,000 deaths on the roads. More than one-quarter of the victims were under fifteen, and more than one-half over sixty-five.[3] More children under fifteen die from such accidents than from any one infectious disease, and of all those children who die between their first and fifth years, home accidents are the third largest cause of death.

J. W. B. Douglas and J. M. Blomfield (*op. cit.*) found that children were particularly liable to have accidents when they were starting to sit up and learning to walk; that boys (under five) had about one-third more accidents than girls and that the boys' accidents were the more serious ones. The children in their survey who had more than one accident were superior in health and physique. In particular their hearing and visual acuity were above average (pp. 85–9). The chief danger periods are washing day, dinner-time and tea-time, for most of the accidents seem to arise from risks inherent in ordinary domestic activities, especially at busy times. For children under six Sunday afternoons, when the parents take a rest, is another danger period.[4]

In 1951, for all ages, falls accounted for fifty-eight per cent of fatal accidents in the home, burns and scalds thirteen per cent,

[1] *Children under Five* (London, 1958), p. 141.
[2] F. A. E. Crew in *B.M.J.* I (1953), 1125.
[3] *Report of the Standing Interdepartmental Committee on Accidents in the Home* (H.M.S.O., 1953), p. 1.
[4] Parliamentary Secretary, Ministry of Transport (*Hansard*, 18 March 1953).

suffocation twelve per cent and coal-gas poisoning eight per cent.[1] No accurate estimate of the number of non-fatal accidents can be made, but from a congested Birmingham area, out of a population of 13,000, the Birmingham Accident Hospital during 1948 treated nine per cent of the children under ten and three per cent of the adults for home accidents. It is extraordinary that local authorities still build houses with no provision for securing a fireguard to an open fire; and extraordinary too that there is still widespread ignorance that parents can be prosecuted for failing to guard fires in the presence of young children.

Lord Amulree, who introduced the Fireguards Bill, said that although the Bill would be of some value in ensuring that electric, gas and other fires would in future be sold with a proper guard, most burns were caused by coal fires.[2] There were 130 fatal burns a year from coal fires, compared with seventy from electric, fifty-three from gas and about fifty-eight from other fires.

Women's and children's clothes in the last half century have become progressively more inflammable.[3] Coroners have repeatedly called attention to the danger of children's flannelette and winceyette garments. Some fabrics can be made fire-resistant but others, such as nylon, may be rendered inflammable by a finishing process. The British Standards Institution Committee Report (May 1957) recommends that a definite 'level of safety' should be established, so that suitable labels may guide the public and the shopkeepers as to the reasonable safety of fabrics which they cannot otherwise judge.

Because there is a much lower death-rate from scalds than from burns, their gravity is often underestimated. Bad kitchen design can create many opportunities for scalding accidents: as a principle, the cooker and sink should be aligned along the same, or at most, adjacent walls. The most serious scalding hazard in the British

[1] Perhaps most of the deaths attributed to suffocation are acute infections wrongly diagnosed and the figure may therefore be unreliable (D. Swinscow in B.M.J. 2 (1951), 1004). A new danger to infants is the plastic bib. Two deaths have been recorded (*The Times*, 16 July 1957) where the infant had dribbled, the plastic bib had stuck to his face and then he had been unable to breathe.

[2] House of Lords, 8 December 1954.

[3] L. Colebrook, V. Colebrook, J. P. Bull and D. M. Jackson in B.M.J. 1 (1956), 1380.

house is perhaps the tea-pot. The risk could be reduced if the lid had two lugs and the base were wide instead of incurved as it usually is. The *British Medical Journal*, when reviewing the report of the Standing Inter-departmental Committee, said: 'A visit to a patient may afford a timely moment for a word of advice on the dangers of an unguarded fire or the hazards of a slipping rug that the doctor himself has barely survived. He can in addition command the patient's attention in a way that no organisation ever can. No poster or pamphlet can match the doctor's personal guidance.'[1] Colebrook has pointed out that it is rare for a second case of severe burns to come from the same home; but this is a painful way for parents and children to learn.[2]

Lord Amulree has also drawn attention to the large number of children who are poisoned accidentally, apparently because so many homes are becoming rather like a chemist's shop.[3] It appears that children are often given dangerous tablets, and sometimes tablets are left lying about. In 1953 169 children died from taking poison by mistake; one-quarter of them under the age of five. It has been reckoned that there is one death in every twenty cases of poisoning, and that roughly eight hundred children each year are being poisoned by mistake. Some propaganda could well be directed towards the education of parents in keeping poisons out of the way of children.

Death from accident as a major cause of mortality is not, of course, peculiar to Britain but is a characteristic of any advanced country. It has been pointed out that according to a Dutch study the rate for violent deaths for pre-school children in England and Wales is lower than any other country, including Canada, Australia, the U.S.A. and all Western European countries for which statistics are available.[4]

The unmarried

The unmarried mother finds some difficulty in providing herself and her child with a home. Very rarely the mother is an older single professional woman who wants to have a baby without the

---

[1] *B.M.J.* **1** (1953), 211.
[2] *Lancet*, **2** (1949), 181.
[3] *Hansard*, 8 December 1954.
[4] *Med. Off.* **94** (1955), 248.

encumbrance of a husband. Even then, however, the child's birth presents her with practical and emotional difficulties not dissimilar from those of other unmarried mothers. The current public attitude to an unmarried mother is very mixed: she is condemned for her wrongdoing, she is pitied for her misfortune, she is thought to be more sinned against than sinning, she is despised for her stupidity. The attitude may be compared with that towards the woman divorcee who has committed adultery. She has broken her vows and deceived her husband, but public opinion condemns her less than the unmarried mother.

The personal problem of the unmarried mother is largely determined by the attitude of her family. She is in need of help and advice from the moment her pregnancy is discovered. She may seek it and find it within her family; perhaps one of the better solutions, though it has many difficulties, is for the child to be reared by his maternal grandmother. But in some families the parents are greatly concerned about the effect upon younger sisters, and in any case there may seem to be an unending series of disclosures to make: to relations, friends, neighbours, employers and officials. The girl may be rejected by her family. Rejection may express itself in the silence of ostracism or the constant nagging of righteousness as well as in the more obvious physical action of throwing the girl out.

The reasons for her pregnancy are rarely simple and the pregnancy itself may well be the symptom of emotional instability. The majority of unmarried mothers have but one irregular pregnancy. Where there are later ones, the girls are either mentally retarded and physically advanced or are of psychopathic personality—and in such cases help is hard to give. Unmarried mothers are suspected to be, in part, victims of their high fertility.[1] Greenland also points out the significance of residence away from home and of occupations that give women a greater opportunity for intimate contact with men.

A girl who is mentally retarded or deficient may be unable to

[1] D. V. Glass and E. Grebenick, *Trend and Pattern of Fertility in Great Britain* (H.M.S.O., 1955); C. Greenland in *Med. Off.* **99** (1958), 265.

manage unaided. It is often advocated that the baby be removed from such a girl as soon as possible. In practice many mentally defective girls make affectionate and attentive mothers (see p. 144). The baby is in need of his mother's care and caring for her child may greatly contribute to the girl's own steadiness and to the maturation of her emotions. The girl is in need of supervision, material security and guidance herself. This is difficult to come by, but if it can be attained both the mother and her infant may do very well. What sort of advice and help she will receive and what sort of agency she will be referred to will largely be determined by the doctor's own outlook, feelings and beliefs. The girl—normal, mentally retarded or psychopathic—is on any count a social casualty. Her chances of building a home are poor.

The discovery of her pregnancy tends to be later rather than earlier. There is always the possibility that she genuinely does not understand her condition. Whether she is in need of explanation or not, she will certainly need some emotional steadying and support. Even the girl who comes for treatment, when the explanation is given, joins the vast majority who have really come to ask the doctor 'What is to happen to me, what can I do?' The diagnosis of pregnancy has confronted the doctor with a patient whose problems are psychiatric and social. The objectives are the social and psychiatric rehabilitation of the girl and the nearest possible approximation to home life for the child.

It is as well to discover, early, whether the girl is simply one of those who will be married when accommodation becomes available or who, for any other reason, may be expected to marry in the ordinary course of events. Delay of marriage until pregnancy is so common that one investigator found it to be the main social influence leading to late attendance among primigravidae at a hospital ante-natal clinic.[1] Even where this may be the case, her reactions and those of her family may still be painful. Most girls who are aware of their condition, it is commonly believed, make some attempt to terminate their pregnancy; a girl coming to the doctor, therefore, will need assurance that she has done neither

[1] R. Illsley in *Med. Off.* **95** (1956), 107.

herself nor her child any injury. She may well need some assurance concerning venereal disease, for she has almost certainly been worried about it. The best way to give assurance is the positive one: to assure her that she, and the future baby, are fit and well—if that is the case. The girl who is living in faithful concubinage with a man may either present herself as an unmarried mother or may disclose the fact that she is not married after she is told of the diagnosis. She may react like the married woman who will adjust herself to a wanted child, or like the married mother of an unwanted child; or her world may collapse, leaving her a pregnant single woman.

The doctor's role is to assist the patient and her family to accept what is inevitable and to make the best possible adjustment. Welfare facilities are available for the mother and her child, exactly as for other mothers, though she may be slow to take advantage of them. The argument is that the health of neither mother nor child should suffer. If she can be persuaded to use these facilities and to adjust her life very much as though she were a widow the best results may be achieved.[1] She is, however, a good deal more vulnerable than the widow and it may be impossible for her to approximate to the normal experience of motherhood.

For the confinement, mother and baby homes are available for the unmarried mother, some statutory, some voluntary and some closely related to adoption agencies. The official attitude of the Ministry of Health is that a mother should be encouraged to keep her child and care for him herself. In many of the mother and baby homes, however, it is assumed that the child will be adopted. The Hurst Committee on Adoption recommended that more time should be given for the mother to decide whether to keep her baby or not.[2] At present the child must be at least six weeks old before the mother can give her formal consent to his adoption, but the child may be placed with the prospective adopters before that. If this is done, of course, the need of a home disappears. About one-third of the mothers take this decision.

[1] But see below, p. 125.
[2] *Report of the Departmental Committee on the Adoption of Children* (H.M.S.O.), pp. 14–15.

At the notification of birth the child's illegitimacy is declared. In order to reduce the social disadvantage of the child there are now 'shortened' birth certificates, without reference to parentage. Whether they effectively shield the child from misfortune when applying for posts—or on the other occasions when a birth certificate is produced—is doubtful. The legal, as distinct from social, disability of the bastard is now, for practical purposes, reduced to matters of inheritance. The first country to abolish the status of illegitimacy was Norway, in 1915,[1] followed by Sweden (1917), Finland (1922), Denmark (1937) and, after the war, Russia, Israel and the States of Dakota and Arizona. Illegitimacy rates have fallen with the spread of the knowledge of contraception in most northern European countries: in Norway, for example, from eight per cent (1915) to five per cent (1954), and in Sweden from fifteen per cent (1917) to nine per cent (1954).

If the mother is to keep the child, she needs special help in creating a home, since she has no husband. Obtaining special help for her is difficult, for it is open to the criticism that it condones the girl's experience and perhaps induces others to do the same. The fact remains, however, that she needs assistance—and on balance more than the widow. Her problem is to create her home single-handed.

The mother may compel the father to contribute to the support of the child. She may also be advised to adopt her own child, in order to avoid future complications. This procedure, which was expressly contemplated in the Adoption Act, 1950, establishes a clear legal relation between the mother and the child and renders it unnecessary for her to simulate married status. She may quite openly retain her status of spinster, thus disposing of all the form-filling and official difficulties. She does not, however, avoid the problem of all adopters: explaining to the child his origin.

If she cannot return to her parents, she will probably do no better than to find a foster-mother for her child or to pay for him to be maintained in a home. Her contact with her child is likely to be no more than at some week-ends. It is next to impossible for a woman with a baby who must go out to work, whether she be unmarried

---

[1] I. Pinchbeck in *Brit. J. Sociol.* 5 (1954), 317.

or a widow, to find a room, or a landlady ready to take her in. Inevitably, if the mother is at work, some at least of the care of the baby, especially in an emergency, will fall upon the landlady. A 'respectable' landlady may well think twice before taking in a girl with an unexplained baby.

The girl's attitude to her baby is bound to be complex and ambivalent and even if she is able to create a home her emotional difficulties are bound to be considerable and sometimes insoluble.

The childless

Some couples create a home but have no children, and they seek to adopt, foster or act as guardians to children. Their services are much sought-after today; but their reasons for offering their services must be understood. Adult attitudes to children are never simple, and socially approved attitudes vary from place to place and time to time. It is important that some care be taken to see that any contrived family will manifest from the start the currently approved attitudes.

Adoption

The reasons adults may have for seeking to adopt a child are not always obvious and not always contributory to the best interests of either child or prospective adopter. The doctor should act in close co-operation with those whose statutory duty it is to ensure the best interests of the child. Not all adoption society workers or local authorities will handle every adoption wisely: but on the whole their greater experience leads to less failures. Furthermore, the arrangement of any adoption entails a responsibility which is better carried by a corporate body—which does not die, or move away, for example—than by an individual.

The simplest situation arises when a couple, for medical or surgical reasons, have no children and desire them. There are many factors relevant to becoming a parent: parents commonly take some pride in possession—the birth of one's first-born is a considerable event—enjoy their feeling of superiority and power over children, realise their child is a joint enterprise, welcome him as a common and more or less permanent interest. They look to the child's future, identifying it with their own: he will carry on the name, tradition, business, have opportunities the parents lacked or failed to realise. Though they may not be able to recite them all, parents have their own standards of conduct, axioms, self-evident assumptions and beliefs, and are more or less irrational and inconsistent in their own behaviour. All these things are brought to bear upon the child. They come to the child from outside him, shaping him, making him his parents' son.

These things, however, are not enough: loving a child involves feeling warmly comfortable towards him, protecting him against harmful forces, serving him, guiding and watching over him while he develops at his own pace in his own way. In educational theory, some emphasise the need to mould and teach, some the need to let the individual flower; but within the home, between parents and child both elements are inevitably present. Today much greater value is placed upon the second element; some firmly believe that it is the 'correct', 'ideal' and 'only' way to rear a child. Be that as it may, present-day parents are, speaking generally, expected to be permissive rather than repressive, easy-going rather than strict, and the couple who by the standards of thirty years ago might have been highly regarded today may be thought to be too strict to be suitable adopters.

There must be reasonable certainty that the adults of the contrived family can supply the approved feelings—not to the exclusion of the others, for that is absurd—but in a manner that determines the whole patterning of their attitude to the child. In practice it is far from easy to tell whether a couple will make suitable adoptive parents. But it is not until the good match of child and adopters has been made—the parents not too old, the child not a mere acquisition nor a desperately-sought link between a couple drifting apart—that the real problems begin.

The child should know he is adopted. The Hurst Committee recommended that parents should be compelled to give an undertaking to the court that they would rear him in that knowledge. Some parents tell even their natural children that they were bought in a shop, or specially chosen at the doctor's, and the child sees the point of choosing him (Jim) and not George next door and commends his parents for their shrewdness. The adopted child must come to realise that he was specially chosen, just as the parents chose each other for a lifelong relationship. The child in due course is bound to ask questions about his natural parents and the questions must be answered. They are no more odd than other people's interests in family trees and parish registers and if all is well with the child in his home there is no undue harm in unearthing the past.

It takes time for the child to belong, however early the adoption, and as new traits—especially disapproved ones—arise, the questions of heredity come up. They must be discussed, together with the reactions of parents and child to the relationship generally, just as similar questions are discussed in families where there is a biological as well as a social bond.

The single adopter has his or her own problems, similar to those of the widowed. The provision of satisfactory physical contacts between child and adult may be difficult and without the assistance of the extended family, within which the child may come to find his place, the child's life may well be emotionally and socially poor.

Adoption orders may be made by the High, county or juvenile courts. The person to be adopted must be under twenty-one and must not have been married. The courts have powers in certain circumstances to dispense with the consent of the child's parents or guardian or those who contribute to its maintenance, which is otherwise statutory. The applicant must be at least twenty-five years old and at least twenty-one years older than the child—unless he is a relative of the child, when he must be at least twenty-one, or is the natural parent of the child. A man as sole applicant is rarely permitted to adopt a female child. A husband and wife—but only a husband and wife—may jointly adopt; one spouse may not adopt without the consent of the other.

An adoption order may be made only if the child has been in the possession of the prospective adopter or adopters for at least the three preceding months, and if the prospective adopter has given notice of at least three months to the local welfare authorities (the county or the county borough council) of an intention to apply. The court appoints a guardian *ad litem*—that is, in the eyes of the law. This is usually the local authority, which acts through the children's officer. An adopted child has the rights of one born in lawful wedlock to the adopters.

Fostering

Fostering is a less committed relationship than adoption and for that reason some of the elements in a parent-child relationship are excluded. Many healthy adults have the best reason to be grateful for the prolonged loving care of a woman other than their mother— and not always of her race and language—during infancy and child-hood: their nurse. The relationship between mother, child and nurse is clear, and includes the element of reward. With foster-parents the relationship is not always so clear. Monetary reward is not permitted: the sole basis is assumed to be the foster-parents' wish and ability to care for children, and payments are estimated only to cover outgoings. The foster-home may be greatly superior by any yardstick to that of the parents, but how to preserve the proper relationship is by no means obvious, and, even when it has been attained, it may well be upset by the parents, so presenting real difficulties to both child and foster-parents.

The regulations concerning foster-parents and other daily child-minders (see p. 137) refer only where there is some monetary payment. Children are sometimes looked after without any payment. This arrangement may sometimes be made for the best possible reasons and produce the happiest results, but occasionally, as when illegitimate children are handed over soon after birth, difficulties may arise. The Curtis Committee drew attention to the danger and Professor Moncrieff has again pointed out the need for some supervision where these informal arrangements are made.[1]

Foster-parents with homes and families of their own prefer, in general, to receive younger children rather than older, long-stay rather than short, girls rather than boys, and normal rather than exceptional children. The supply of foster-parents falls short of the

[1] *Child Health and the State* (Oxford, 1953), p. 41.

demand; it may be that while there is a shortage of boarding-out officers in the employ of local authorities some suitable families remain undiscovered.

Fostering: single women

While it is probable that the overwhelming majority of women who are capable of giving children what they need are early appropriated by men and care, to the satisfaction of everyone, for the children of their union, there may be the best of reasons why a woman is single, and childless. Although in some cases her unmarried state may be due to some defect, she may yet be capable of bringing to children the approved attitudes and making them happy. It is apparent, however, that, if only in order to know what is to be provided for the child, the reasons for a single woman's offering her services as an adopter, foster-mother or worker in a children's home must be understood.

The element of reward is frankly recognised in the family group home (see p. 140). The house mother there may be married and her husband employed elsewhere. In the grouped cottage homes and large institutional homes, the female staff is for the most part unmarried. The married male staff in these large homes, however devoted, have their independent family lives.

The disturbed or broken

Home life may be disturbed in its function in five main ways by: (1) the nature of the occupation or way of life of the parents; (2) the incapacitation by illness or accident of the parent; (3) quarrelling; (4) separation or divorce; (5) death of one or both parents.

(1) *Parental way of life*

It is possible for the home to function without one of the spouses, or with one spouse away from home for long periods, as all acquainted with seafaring, service, diplomatic, colonial and missionary families know. Families who work in fairgrounds, circuses, canals and on the stage suffer the disadvantage of being constantly on the move, as do the families of some of the very rich. Some occupations which demand irregular hours or shift work make the organisation of the home difficult. Parents cannot be regularly available to meet their children's needs and may of necessity be sleeping at any time of the day. Families in which either or both parents are employed in transport are perhaps the commonest example.

(2) Parental incapacity

Illness or accident may disturb the family immediately, and the result may continue or become permanent. The incapacity of the husband may bring financial anxiety, added demand on the wife's energies, and a reorganisation of the household routine; but on balance, it is probably less serious than that of the wife, except in the now rare household in which she has few or no domestic duties. The removal of the wife and mother may easily create a situation where there is no longer a family, with its home, but merely people in a dwelling for whom there is no one to clean, to cook, to look after the children and to do the negotiations at the door.

(3) Quarrelling parents

Parents are apt during the emotional stress of quarrels or of bereavement to underestimate the difficulties of maintaining their homes without their partners: to overestimate their own ability to combine two functions, and that of their extended family to support them. Quarrelling and unhappy couples may be referred to the Marriage Guidance Council.[1] Through the voluntary services of selected counsellors, the Council gives advice to engaged couples on the mental, spiritual and physical aspects of marriage as well as advising couples who are unhappy or are in conflict in marriage. The Catholic organisation is called the Catholic Marriage Advisory Council.

Many working-class couples seek advice initially from the probation officers at the local courts. The officers are well placed to

[1] See G. B. Carruthers in *B.M.J.* I (1956), 1478.

advise and refer cases to social work agencies. They can also assist either party to begin legal action, if necessary.

Couples may consult the case-working agencies, some of which make special provision for this work. The Family Welfare Association is the main body in this country engaged in family case work. It believes that the welfare of the community depends upon the maintenance of family life and the preservation of personal independence. Its work consists in case work designed to reinstate the temporary social casualty and also in the formation of public opinion about new social legislation. It co-operates with government departments, local authorities, hospitals, schools and many voluntary bodies.

(4) *Separation and divorce*

When difficulties arise between couples their own notions of marriage are brought up against those of the law—and the law itself is now being questioned. There are two forms of marriage, both, now, subject to the law—the religious and the civil. For many, the religious service creates an indissoluble bond. Liberal churchmen, however, approve divorce on the ground of charity, as a desperate remedy for an incurable evil; but they do not accept that divorce can be by consent, for marriage is not any ordinary contract. The civil marriage can be broken only if there is a matrimonial offence. The Royal Commission on Marriage and Divorce was appointed because in 1951 the Commons gave a second reading to a Bill which would have admitted seven years *de facto* separation as a ground for divorce and would thus have introduced an entirely new principle.

Divorce and children. The need to provide children with a warm and stable atmosphere is now everywhere acknowledged. When the couple find that their personal happiness, their love—the basis of their marriage, as they believe, and the basis of their children's healthy development—is gone, they are faced with an extremely difficult situation. On the one hand they have their duty to provide their children with this very happiness which they themselves have lost; on the other, their partnership can be broken only by a matrimonial offence, if at all. The notion of the necessity for divorce of a matrimonial offence persists, however; so much so that in the report of the Morton Commission one of the few recommendations that were unanimous was that the 'injured' party should be free to choose between divorce and permanent judicial separation even though the decision be founded on malice and contrary to the general interest.[1]

The Commission fell back on the need for preparation for marriage:

> We are convinced that the real remedy for the present situation lies in other directions: in fostering in the individual the will to do his duty by the community; in strengthening his resolution to make marriage a union for life; in inculcating a proper sense of responsibility towards his children. These objectives can only be achieved by education in the widest sense, by specific instruction before marriage, and by providing facilities for guidance after marriage and for reconciliation if breakdown threatens.

When the couple divorce the innocent party has custody of the children. For some time a welfare officer has been attached to the Divorce Division of the High Court, to supervise the arrangements made for the care of the children of broken marriages. Welfare officers are now to be appointed in all the forty-two towns in England, Scotland and Wales which have Divorce Courts. The law now requires that no decree of divorce or judicial separation be made final until the court is satisfied that, as far as is practicable, adequate arrangements have been made for the future of the children.

The mother has a right, as the father has, to apply to the court in respect of any matter affecting the infant's upbringing or property. The court's power to make an order for custody and access may be exercised although the mother is living with the father; the court may also order the father to pay towards the child's maintenance. The paramount consideration, in law, is the welfare of the child and not the enforcement of the father's traditional rights.

Maintenance. The rights and duties of husbands and wives towards each other and towards their children are enforceable by law.

---

[1] *Report of the Royal Commission on Marriage and Divorce* (H.M.S.O. 1956).

When one or other deserts, or fails to maintain, the remaining spouse may obtain a court order. Couples may also separate by agreement—most prudently with a document drawn up by a solicitor.

When the woman proceeds in the magistrates' court against her husband she applies for maintenance for herself and her children on an assessment made by the magistrate. The husband's payments may, if necessary, be made at the court and collected there by the wife. The husband may be directed not to molest either wife or children. An order may be granted upon the application of a married woman for aggravated assault, adultery, desertion, wilful neglect to provide reasonable maintenance, persistent cruelty to her or her infant children, habitual drunkenness or drug-taking, insistence upon sexual intercourse whilst knowingly suffering from venereal disease, and compulsion by her husband to submit to prostitution.

An application may be made by a husband on the grounds of adultery, habitual drunkenness or drug-taking or persistent cruelty to his children. In Scotland a spouse may obtain judicial separation only on the grounds of adultery or cruelty or habitual drunkenness. The husband, in Scotland, is generally liable to aliment his wife: provide her with bed and board.

(5) *Death*

When either parent dies, there is a natural tendency for the survivor to return to his or her parents with the children of the marriage. The success of this solution depends upon the availability of accommodation and upon the relationship between the widowed spouse and the parents.

Working-class difficulties. It is difficult for a working-class widow to keep her home going for, obliged as she will be to go to work, it calls for great physical exertion. It is almost impossible for a working-class widower to keep his home going, unless he can depend upon the extended family; a housekeeper is difficult to find and expensive and she can scarcely live in; he is more or less compelled to marry again to maintain his home.

Middle-class difficulties. The better-off widower is not so badly placed, even if he is without an extended family to call upon, since he can afford to hire a nanny and housekeeper and can send the older children to boarding school. But if he is alone, however much money he has, his difficulties are still considerable. Domestic staff have their hours of duty, their days off and their holidays; they fall sick and they change their jobs. School holidays are long. If the children are to enjoy something like normal home life, most of his non-working hours, at least, must for some years, be devoted to the children. It is not particularly easy for him to mother his son, nor is he likely to be skilful in giving his daughter the feminine values which he admired in his wife.

The middle-class widow who can afford servants and is not compelled to work to provide an income may manage better: but again, if she is to be a good parent, she has the work of two to do, will be much tied by her children, and will find herself unable to father her daughter or to give her son the masculine values which she admired in her husband.

Guardianship. On the death of one parent, the other may be the sole guardian if the dead parent has not appointed one, or the court may, if it thinks fit, appoint a guardian or guardians to act jointly with the survivor. If a guardian considers the surviving parent unfit to have the custody of the child he may apply to the court, which may either order the guardian to act jointly with the parent or give him sole custody while granting right of access to the child by the parent. The court may also order the parent to pay the guardian for the child's maintenance. A court of summary juris-diction may deal with applications, not necessarily in open court; but they may not award payment of sums exceeding £1 a week towards the maintenance of a person under twenty-one and they cannot deal with questions of property.

The term 'wards of court' is used for minors who are brought under the authority of the court by an application to it on their behalf, even though no guardian is appointed—although perhaps strictly it should apply only to a person under the care of a guardian formally appointed by the court.

Parents and guardians of children entitled to property on coming of age act within the wide jurisdiction of the court, which will dismiss guardians who have acted dishonestly, unfairly or improperly towards their wards and compel them to account for the rents and profits of the minor's estates. The court may, in disputes, direct the manner in which the ward is to be educated and maintained to the extent of naming the school and the university he will attend. The marriage of a ward, whether male or female, must be with the consent of the court.

Widows' cash benefits. There are certain cash benefits for any widow, providing that her husband had paid at least 156 national insurance contributions before his death. If payments are to be made at the full rate the husband must have had a yearly average of fifty contributions or credits. The widow's allowance is paid for thirteen weeks after the husband's death; there is in addition a payment for each child—widowed mother's allowance—which continues during widowhood or until the children are beyond the qualifying age. The widow's pension is paid immediately after the widow's allowance comes to an end, provided that she has been married for at least ten years and is between fifty and sixty at the time of her husband's death. It may also be paid when the widowed mother's allowance ends because the children are beyond the qualifying age if she is then over forty and ten years have elapsed since her marriage. The pension may also be paid temporarily during illness. There are deductions for earnings. All else failing, she must fall back on National Assistance.[1]

Facilities for the disturbed or broken home

At any time, the disturbed home may need the services of the home nurse and the home help (see p. 115), of the national insurance office or of the national assistance officer. If legal advice is necessary and beyond the family's means, it is available in most towns through Legal Advice Bureaux.

---

[1] Investigations into widowhood are rare, but for an account of London widows and their difficulties see P. Marris, *Widows and their Families* (London, 1958).

Special categories. Where there is physical separation of the parents because of their way of life, some facilities are usually available to support family life. The churches have their own provisions for the families of those in their service. For servicemen, the two largest agencies are the Forces Help Society and the Soldiers', Sailors' and Airmen's Family Association. These are voluntary bodies, giving assistance in cases of emergency and special distress not covered by government schemes to families of all members of the forces and the widows and orphans of those deceased.

Day nursery. The day nursery or the nursery school may give some assistance in maintaining the home as a going concern. The nurseries are designed to care for children under school age whose mothers are obliged to go out to work; they do not provide any formal education. The schools, normally, admit children from two to five years of age, and the aim is mainly educational. Day nurseries are provided by the local maternity and child welfare authority, nursery schools by the local education authority; both may be provided by voluntary organisations. The number of day nurseries rose to 1560 during the war but was in 1956 reduced to some 530. The majority of admissions to day nurseries are 'priority cases'. It is possible that regular attendance there may give a sense of order and security to a small child's life that might otherwise be lacking. The importance of mothering young children in nurseries is now understood.

Child minders. By the Nurseries and Child Minders Regulation Act (1948) it is an offence for premises to be used as a day nursery without being registered with the local health authority (the county or county borough council) or for a daily child minder to take for reward three or more children under five, not relatives, from more than one household, without registration. The Act also empowers local health authorities to impose requirements, in connection with registration, concerning the maximum number of children to be received, and in the case of day nurseries, the number and qualifications of staff, the provision of suitable food, etc.

The Ministries of Health and Education in 1945 pointed out that provision might be made by local authorities for the occasional care of children under school age, whether or not their mothers go out to work, so that the mothers may have reasonable opportunity for rest and recreation away from their homes and children. As important as the nursery schools are the holiday homes, generally run by voluntary societies, but receiving a local authority subvention, where a mother and her infant or young children may have a recuperative holiday.

Private boarding out. The infant life protection provisions of the Public Health Act 1936 as amended by the Children Act 1948 require that notice be given to the welfare authority by any person except a relative or legal guardian who undertakes for reward the nursing and maintenance of a child under school-leaving age apart from its parents. Anyone receiving the Family or Guardians Allowance is deemed to maintain the child for reward: the term 'reward' need not imply any element of profit.

The education authority may assist in sending a child to boarding school, for it is bound to provide residential education for children when it is in the interests of the child to do so.

Immediate succour. Catastrophe may come to a home by way of accident, illness, death or a sudden quarrel. The children may be in need of immediate succour. This is ordinarily forthcoming from neighbours, relatives or through the police and the official channels. An allowance is payable to any person in whose family an orphan child is included, if one of its parents was an insured person under the National Insurance Act. An allowance may be paid in certain circumstances when the child has been adopted or is illegitimate or where the parents are divorced or one parent cannot be traced.

Local authority. There is a duty laid on the county councils and county borough councils under the Children Act to receive into care any child under seventeen who has neither parent nor guardian, or is abandoned by them or is lost; whose parents or guardian are temporarily or permanently prevented by illness, incapacity, or any other circumstances from providing for his proper accommodation, maintenance and upbringing and where the intervention of the local authority is necessary in the interests of the welfare of the child. Children may be taken into care on application by parents or guardian who are temporarily unable to look after them.

The local authority must appoint a Children's Committee and a Children's Officer. Upon receiving a child into care the authority has a duty to keep him in care, if necessary, till he is eighteen, subject to the consent of the parent or parents. It has a parallel duty, however, to make sure that the child's care is taken over as soon as practicable by the parents, guardian, relatives or friends. The authority may relinquish its responsibility for the child under various circumstances: care may be taken over by another local authority, or, in the case of a war orphan, by the Minister of Pensions, or the child may become subject to the Mental Deficiency or Lunacy Acts or to an approved school order. The number of children in care is fairly stable at about 62,000. Every year about 39,000 come into care and as many go out. About forty-five per cent are boarded out.

Reception centres. It was a recommendation of the Curtis Report[1] that every authority should establish at least one Reception Centre in its area for children deprived of normal home life, there to make the immediate provision necessary and to investigate the long-term needs. Opinion has been sharply divided as to their usefulness: indeed, some consider them to be dangerous.

The local authority must exercise its powers so as to further the child's best interests and enable him to achieve the proper development of his character and abilities. It is required to board out children in homes that it has inspected and approved; the children's home is to be used only where it is impracticable or undesirable to board out. Boarding out is not a simple matter. It is easier to place girls than boys, younger rather than the older children, the normal rather than the abnormal, the long-term rather than the short-term. The payment covers only maintenance to exclude the profit motive. Foster-parents, we have seen, do not long tolerate contact between the child and his parents; they are often unable, even if willing, to accept several children of one

[1] *Report of the Committee on the Care of Children* (H.M.S.O. 1946), pp. 10–11.

family; and they tend to be severer in their judgment of the fostered child's conduct than in that of their own. Where boarding-out is either not possible or impracticable, the child may be placed in a children's home, of which there are three main sorts.

Family group homes are particularly designed to keep brothers and sisters together but are also used for other children who are not boarded out. These homes are more or less ordinary houses, accommodating up to a dozen children; there is a resident married couple, the wife being the employee of the local authority, and the children live a life in the neighbourhood closely approximating to that of a normal family. The medical care is arranged in co-operation with the medical officer of health or local family doctors.

Grouped cottage homes. Grouped cottage homes, each home containing ten to twenty children under the charge of a male superintendent, are segregated societies, but were a considerable advance in their day. Most children there now go out to the ordinary school and sex segregation is not usual. Every opportunity is needed to integrate the children into the life of the neighbourhood. This is by no means easy; but the need for it, and sometimes the opportunity, will be plain to the visiting medical officer.

Large homes. Large homes may vary in size from those providing for forty or so children to those which house several hundred. The staff do not necessarily move with the times.[1] Children's homes provided by voluntary organisation must be registered with the Secretary of State.

Residential nurseries. Children under five who cannot be placed in a family group home or boarded out are placed in residential nurseries.

Hostels. Regulations require that hostels or lodgings be provided for children who have been in care and are now over school age and under twenty-one. Little has in fact been done to provide them, but practically all organisations which have children in care have some system of 'after-care'.

[1] See D. Ford, *The Deprived Child* (London, 1955).

Parental rights. The authority may, by resolution, assume parental rights in respect of the child; they must notify parents (if any) or guardian, who may object—in which case the resolution lapses until a court, on application by the local authority, decides the case.

Ineffective

Families may be ineffective because of a defect in one or both parents. These are the 'problem families'. The defect may manifest itself as cruelty to the children, or neglect, or a general squalid incompetence.

The *Oxford English Dictionary* defines cruelty as 'a disposition to inflict suffering; delight in or indifference to another's pain'. Cruelty to and neglect of children are punishable. The same authority gives 'neglect' as 'failing to bestow the proper care and attention upon'. What is or is not considered cruelty to or neglect of a child will change as public standards change. J. B. Priestley, in the introduction to *The Neglected Child in the Family*,[1] noted that this report makes no mention of those children surrounded by all the luxuries who are left so emotionally insecure that they grow up anti-social. The family doctor does well to keep his eye on all exceptional homes: those where the parents are very rich or very distinguished, or adhere to minority ways.

It is not cruel to take a knife to the infant boy and circumcise him; not cruel to hold down the shrinking child and cover his face with the anaesthetising mask; not cruel to remove a frightened and ill child from his home and parents and to isolate him in hospital; not cruel to nag a child, not neglectful to omit any sexual instruction.

Detection

Family squalor and incompetence cannot always be recognised in the consulting room; but the facts declare themselves at a home visit. Cruelty does not always make itself plain at either place. The doctor when examining the child may well be the first to discover the signs of physical maltreatment. Even so, he may not

---

[1] Oxford University Press, 1948.

always be sufficiently certain of himself to accuse the mother, nor indeed may he know what to do next, whether she confirms or denies the maltreatment. But personal responsibility cannot be avoided. In March 1956 a child of two was starved for the second time in his own home to the point where he was desperately ill, unconscious and grossly wasted. When, for the second time, he was taken to hospital, he died. How the child's condition escaped every experienced eye is not understood.

The Children and Young Persons (Amendment) Act, 1952, imposed a duty upon the local authority to investigate any allegation of neglect brought to its notice. But many people still prefer to refer cases of suspected cruelty to the local inspector of the National Society for the Prevention of Cruelty to Children. He has the advantage of being expert, and, while recognised, at the same time unofficial.

Neighbours, teachers, welfare workers, the police, as well as medical practitioners, solicit his aid. Nevertheless prosecution is not the major part of the Society's work. It is a voluntary society for the prevention of ill-treatment, wrongful neglect, or improper employment of children; also of all conduct by which life, limb or health is wilfully endangered or sacrificed, or by which morals are imperilled or depraved. Officers are appointed who investigate cases about which complaint has been made, and if the accusation is true, parents or guardians are warned and constantly supervised; if warnings are neglected, they are prosecuted by the Society. Prosecution is not resorted to until all other methods of improving the condition of the children have failed.

The gross forms of physical maltreatment of children today are rare and the detection rate is probably high. It has been reported by a joint committee of the B.M.A. and the Magistrates' Association that the figures for 1933, 1948 and 1952 show that an average of rather less than 100,000 children were under the supervision of the N.S.P.C.C. each year.[1] The figures for convictions, however, give a better indication of the proportion of gross cruelty. The number of males imprisoned for cruelty and neglect rose from

[1] *Cruelty to and Neglect of Children* (B.M.A., 1956).

176 in 1933 to a peak of 214 in 1948, and fell to 184 in 1952. The number of females reached a peak of 510 during the war but has since approximated very closely to the figures for male prisoners.

The report observes that cruelty can be more often attributed to emotional instability than to intellectual defect. It maintains that it is often a mistake to give a second chance to the psychopathic and that psychiatric treatment is seldom effective with such people, although the neurotic may be helped.

A short report on thirty-two men and seven women sent to prison in 1954 for cruelty to children drew attention to the fact that violent parents were not as co-operative as neglectful ones and recommended that in all cases there be a remand for psychiatric investigation before the court made its decision.[1]

Neglect

For women who have been convicted of neglect three residential courses have been evolved to which they may be sent under a probation order: one at Plymouth run by the Salvation Army, one at York (formerly at Harrogate) run by the Society of Friends, and a third at Brentwood (Cheshire). Women are now also received voluntarily. The homes are not used to capacity. Mother-craft teaching is now introduced into women's jails—for example at the Winson Green Jail, Birmingham.

M. D. Sheridan has reported on some aspects of the Harrogate scheme.[2] This accepts women with some permanent dwelling who have sufficient intelligence—in the opinion of the medical officer—to benefit from the training. Her ability is assessed at the medical examination before admission, and her general understanding and behaviour during the trial is taken into account. Children under five may accompany the mother. Only women convicted of wilful neglect and not of actual cruelty are eligible. Epileptic, infectious and women known to be pregnant are excluded.

[1] T. C. N. Gibbens and A. Walker, *Cruel Parents* (London, 1956).
[2] In *B.M.J.* I (1956), 91.

The age range of those reported upon was from 17–46 years and their average I.Q. was 79·8. 'At first sight it seems incredible that women possessing such defective intelligence as those representing the lower end of the curve have remained in the ordinary community.' They were found, however, to be 'temperamentally stable, . . . gentle, friendly, contented, and teachable. . . affectionate mothers and faithful wives but thoroughly incompetent housekeepers'. They might manage with one or two children; with more they are overwhelmed.

There was also a small group at the upper end of the intelligence distribution who were found to be invariably unstable and unpredictable in their emotions and behaviour. They appeared to be unable to learn from experience and did not appreciate either the socially unacceptable nature of their actions or omissions or their possible results. Both groups, as well as those in between, contained women 'of moral apathy that is not culpable, of a mental withdrawal which is not schizophrenic, of a physical lethargy which is not mere sloth. It somewhat resembles the dazed inertia of severe physical or mental shock. It is possibly due to malnutrition or to the dulling effect of the repeated assault of adverse circumstance.' The number known to have conceived a child before marriage is some three times the figure for illegitimate and pre-marital conceptions for the general population of married women between sixteen and twenty-four in the years 1946–50.

Seventy-six of the mothers have derived noticeable benefit from the training, twenty-four have failed, usually after initial improvement.

Incompetence

Problem families stand out from the rest today in a way that was impossible a century ago, as both the standard of living and the estimation of the importance of the child have risen.

The punishment of the parent or parents does not always produce a new competence in them; and often their incompetence, though causing concern, may not be enough to merit prosecution. These families, of course, are not peculiar to Britain. A. Querido for example, has described identical ones in the Netherlands.[1] He classified them into:

(i) The 'conditional social' group where a sharply defined cause could be indicated that could be considered as having brought the social debacle about; this might be illness, a combination of unlucky circumstances, etc.

(ii) The 'conditional unsocial' group where a combination of aberrations and maladjustments, together with unfavourable conditions, had brought failure; but under special circumstances such families might be put on their feet again.

(iii) The 'unconditional unsocial' group where there are combinations of personalities and attitudes of such unfavourable character that, even under the most advantageous conditions, the family cannot maintain itself.

Difficulties of housing authorities

Housing authorities find themselves in difficulties with incompetent families. They live in dirt and muddle and fall into arrears with their rent. They fall hopelessly in debt and are evicted. What is to happen then? They come into the care of the social welfare authority. Are they to be put up rent-free? For how long? And where? There comes a time when either the family must be broken up or an effort must be made to see whether the couple can be trained to make a home a more or less going concern. Local authorities prefer, understandably, to work with these families as quietly as possible. The London County Council has indicated that it has a fairly satisfactory scheme by which clusters of houses are put aside for this purpose and supervision is given, particularly at rent-collecting time; a welfare worker befriends the family and assists with budgeting and shopping and advises on running the home. Bristol, it is reported, scatters these families throughout its area in reconditioned houses, but providing a similar supervision.[2] By spreading the families out, they hope to help them achieve a new start and conform to local norms. The methods used are as old as

[1] Med. Off. **75** (1956), 193.
[2] R. C. Wofinden in Med. Off. **94** (1955), 384.

Octavia Hill, but not necessarily any the worse for that. The medical officer of health for Chesterfield takes the view that about fifty of Chesterfield's rural district council's 5000 tenants are 'incorrigible problem families' who should be housed in austerity houses to keep them away from the good-standard tenants. Plans for such houses, it is reported, were rejected by the Ministry of Housing. An insight is given into the official attitude to the problem by the report concerned with the general problem families must face when moved from slum clearance areas.[1] The needs of the individual families must be studied and an attempt made to meet them. It reminds local authorities, for example, that they have powers under the Housing Act to provide essential furniture and bedding for families with low incomes, that families should be given the fullest information, before being moved, about what is going to be done, why it is going to be done, and when. Provision for children's play should be part of the housing scheme and steps should be taken to enable tenants to continue their hobbies and retain their pets. Case-work rather than compulsion is the approach.

The doctor's difficulties

Part of the doctor's difficulties in dealing with these families is that he finds that although every welfare agency has already tried its hand with them, yet even so the problem is rarely recognised early enough for effective rehabilitation. If they were recognised, say, by the health visitor at the birth of the first or second child, there would be an opportunity of preventing difficulties from arising. Whether there is enough adequately trained staff to undertake the work is, however, another matter.

Local authorities are now urged by a joint circular from the Ministries of Health and Education and the Home Office to designate one officer to co-ordinate statutory and voluntary authorities concerned with the care of children in their own homes. Case conferences are called from time to time by the designated officer— sometimes the children's officer, sometimes the medical officer— to co-ordinate action in individual cases.

[1] *Moving from the Slums* (H.M.S.O. 1956).

Mrs Geoffrey Fisher has written of the 'small army of officials and home visitors' who may descend on the family in distress.[1] Subsequently Professor Banks has calculated that there are no fewer than forty people in any given area who may have the right and in some cases the duty of visiting the home on some aspect of social welfare.[2] The subsequent 'overlap' is wasteful of time and energy and is often inefficient. It arises in part from the piecemeal growth of the statutory services and in part from the great array of voluntary services which are a characteristic of British life. There has been a growing understanding of the need to treat the family as a whole.

Family as unit

The formulation of a social problem in terms of families rather than individuals is comparatively new. Hitherto, where the notion has entered British administration its reception has been hostile—as, for example, in the case of the means test, which took into account family income in assessing the amount to be paid to the unemployed when insurance rights were exhausted. Among those rights was included that of the married man to draw amounts in respect of his wife and children. Nevertheless it is true to say that the delinquent or sick child, the wayward adolescent, the neglectful parent has been treated first as an individual and only secondly as a member of a group. Services were given directly to the individual in need. The Family Allowances Act pointed the way to a different attitude, for payment was there made as of right to the mother; and British interest has turned to the French system of assistance, where money is saved or contributed to a family purse instead of a specific service being supplied to an individual.

Family Service Unit

Social thinking has returned to a dictum of John Burns, 'First concentrate on the mother', and commends the Family Service Unit approach. The case-load is necessarily small, for the members

[1] *The Times*, 16 March 1955.
[2] Quoted in *Cruelty to and Neglect of Children*.

enter into the social life of the problem family, perhaps assisting with cooking or cleaning in the home, thus removing the back-log of despair and easing the immediate burdens, for example, of the mother who is overwhelmed by her own incompetence, and at the same time unobtrusively teaching her 'on the job' more efficient ways. The problem of the family is seen as a whole and the object is to increase the members' understanding of the cause of their difficulties and to assist them, in so far as it is possible, to solve them.

Estimates of the number of families in need of their service vary between 40,000 and 80,000.[1] The Units are established in eleven provincial towns and cities and in seven metropolitan boroughs. The Home Office has provided grant aid to local authorities who establish similar services or who delegate the task to the Service Units. The Ministry of Health has recommended the use of health visitors and home helps for the rehabilitation of problem families.

The problem is by no means a simple one. The Home Secretary has appointed a Committee under Lord Ingleby to consider whether local authorities should be given new powers and duties to prevent or forestall the suffering of children through neglect in their own homes (see also p. 83).

Children from incompetent families

It would be wrong to assume that all children of incompetent families are necessarily damaged. A report on the Kent Reception Centre describes the five hundred children sent there between 1947–50.[2] Children of problem families were among the more normal in the Centre. They seldom demanded affection; they were loving and loyal to their incompetent parents and to their siblings, mature and responsible in their attitudes, practical, resourceful and even protective, and they were able to adjust to civilised living. C. H. Wright, on the other hand, has shown, however, concerning a small series of older problem children, that the families may perpetuate themselves.[3] It was found that of thirty-nine marriages

---

[1] *Family Service Units—Eighth Annual Report* (London, 1956).
[2] H. Lewis, *Deprived Children* (Oxford, 1954), pp. 80–1.
[3] C. H. Wright in *Med. Off.* **94** (1955), 381.

contracted by the older children of problem families which were under observation, only nine were known or supposed to be satisfactory, sixteen were unsatisfactory and five had already broken down.

In 1954 the Minister of Health asked local health authorities to see what they could do to prevent this perpetuation. J. A. Scott reported that in London there appeared to be 3022 potential and hard-core problem families.[1] Of these 2456 had a child or children under 5; 526 had children above that age, and forty were in welfare institutions. The percentage prevalence in the County, of these families where there were children under five was 1·43. 'An analysis of aetiological factors in 1000 families revealed emotional instability in 54·5% of the potential and 71·6% of the hard-core problem families; low intelligence or mental deficiency in 42·2 and 67·3% respectively; known or suspected cruelty or neglect in 34·6 and 77·1%; overcrowding or intolerable housing conditions in 44·3 and 60·2%; failure to take advantage of help and services proferred in 30·4 and 51·0%.'

[1] *Lancet*, I (1958), 204.

CHAPTER VIII

THE INFANT AT HOME

MATERNITY AND CHILD WELFARE SERVICES

'The present child welfare services', wrote Sir Leonard Parsons in 1952,

would probably never have arisen if in years gone by general practitioners as a class had taken a real interest in the care of infants and children. This lack of interest may have been due to the fact that rarely was the subject properly presented to medical students:...only too often the mother's request for guidance from the family practitioner as to how to bring up her child remained unanswered, although if the child contracted an illness the attention was frequently beyond criticism.[1]

The Maternity and Child Welfare Act (1918) led to the establishment under the local authorities of a whole-time medical service, the members of which were concerned solely with preventive medicine and were debarred from curative medicine. By 1894 in France Pierre Budin had introduced the 'consultations de nourissons' and Variot and Leon Dufours had opened the 'gouttes de lait' milk depot at which advice was given on artificial feeding. In Belgium, emphasis was laid upon teaching mothers child care: the 'schools for mothers' movement began there. In England, a system of volunteer house-to-house visiting had been instituted.

All four of these notions are present in the contemporary welfare centres; all, with the exception of the 'schools for mothers' idea have developed and adapted themselves to changed conditions. Until 1929 the welfare centres were subject to the supervision of the Board of Education, but by the Local Government Act of that year they were transferred to the Ministry of Health; under neither, however, has the education programme developed as much as

---

[1] Introduction to A. Moncrieff and W. A. R. Thomson (eds.), *Child Health* (Practitioner Handbooks, London, 1952).

welfare workers—or, apparently mothers—would desire. One consequence is that mothers continue to administer medicaments without medical advice. There is little information on the subject, but inquiries made through the health visitors in Bolton in 1953[1] showed that there at least most of the medicaments were of very doubtful therapeutic value: the conclusion was that a great deal of teaching on the normal development of the child was necessary. In particular, doctors and health visitors needed to correct the misconceptions of mothers about the physiological functions of the gastro-intestinal tract and the normal appearance of an infant's mouth. The investigator regarded it as a matter of concern that, in spite of the medicament, 8·6 per cent of the infants were receiving no Vitamin A and D in addition to that contained in their diet.

A relatively new development is the use of ante-natal clinics for psychiatric consultation, to assist the expectant mother to resolve her anxieties and to grow out of her feelings of inadequacy, and there are sometimes similar opportunities in the lying-in wards. These approaches are particularly hopeful, for so many difficulties of the mother and child arise from the success or failure of the earliest relationship. Motherhood education is becoming more important because fewer mothers have had experience of infants in their parental homes during adolescence today than in the past. This is a direct result of smaller households and the fact that families now contain fewer children, born closer together. Anxiety arises from inexperience, the increased demand for parental efficiency, and conflicting advice.

D. P. Lambert has analysed one hundred cases where the chief reason mothers consulted the clinic doctor was mental distress.[2] Eighty-one children were under one year old and in this group the diagnosis in thirty-seven cases was simple anxiety. 'A natural and wholly praiseworthy impulse to do one's best sometimes creates doubt, doubt brings fear, and fear conjures images of horror out of nothing at all.... Often the mothers apologise for taking up

[1] H. Bryant in *Med. Off.* 94 (1955), 209.
[2] D. P. Lambert in *Med. Off.* 94 (1955), 299.

one's time with trifles, and have to be confirmed in the belief that a child welfare centre is a place where trifles can be spoken about without being laughed at.'

Administration of child welfare services

Today the local health authority is responsible for, among other things, the care of expectant and nursing mothers and of children under school age, including dental care, the operation of a service of midwives and health visitors and the provision of home nursing where required.

Hospitals which have children's departments conduct maternity and child welfare centres; the maternity hospitals are responsible for ante-natal and post-natal clinics for the benefit of women who are attended by the hospital doctors during childbirth.

General practitioners may be engaged on a sessional basis at child welfare clinics by the local health authority. Doctors who conduct welfare clinics on their own premises may receive the assistance of the health visitor of the local authority. By these two means a link is established between the local authority service and the general practitioner. The need for this link has been more necessary since the establishment of the Health Service, for wives and young children (who were not covered by the former insurance schemes) now come under the doctor's care, particularly in working class districts, in a way that was formerly not possible. According to a note in the *British Medical Journal*:

About 180 general practitioners are employed by the London County Council on a sessional basis. About sixty-five of these work in the school health service, and the remainder are employed at ante- and post-natal clinics, child welfare centres, vaccination and immunisation clinics, and at dental clinics as anaesthetists. On an average these general practitioners attend two sessions a week each, and are responsible for about one-third of all the sessions worked under the National Health Service Act.[1]

The link is the more needed in ante-natal work because it is accepted that the minimum requirements under the National Health Act— examinations at booking and at the 36th week—are inadequate.[2]

[1] *B.M.J.* I (1953), 1089.   [2] *B.M.J.* I (1956), 1415.

Ante- and post-natal centres attend to the specific health problems of the expectant and nursing mother, and may also provide explanation of the physical processes involved, instruction in exercises and relaxation, and in the conduct of labour. The function of the infant welfare centres is mainly to supervise and instruct mothers in mothercraft; treatment of sick children is not one of their functions. Foods are supplied, when necessary, at cost price or free. They may also assist in the distribution of clothing, maternity outfits, and so on in necessitous cases. The medical officer at the welfare centre satisfies himself that the mother fully understands how to feed, clean, clothe and generally care for her baby until the next interview. The rest of the staff assist her to carry out what she has learnt.

There is no way of ensuring that all mothers secure ante-natal advice. Doubts have been expressed as to how far the original goals of the ante-natal movement have been achieved.[1] These were the removal of anxiety and dread, removing discomfort, ensuring early treatment of complications; increasing the proportion of normal labours, and the lowering of the maternal death and stillbirth rates.

There has been, of course, an enormous reduction in both infant and maternal mortalities and of stillbirths throughout the country. Yet mortality rates differ markedly throughout the country. The rates in Greater London and south-east England for example, compare favourably with the relatively low mortality achieved in the Netherlands and New Zealand,[2] but the rate mounts in the large industrial towns. The lead of the well-to-do families is maintained despite the relatively greater number of primigravidae and the generally higher age of maternity.

In spite of the tremendous reduction in infant mortality during the past thirty years,[3] there has been no narrowing of the differences between the various social classes. This is also true of the stillbirth and neo-natal mortality rates, but less markedly so. J. M. Morris

[1] *Maternity in Great Britain* (Oxford, 1948), p. 22 and quoting F. J. Browne, *Lancet* 2 (1932), 1.
[2] *Neonatal Mortality* (Ministry of Health Report on Public Health and Medical Subjects, 94, H.M.S.O. 1949).
[3] W. P. D. Logan, *Brit. J. Prev. Social Med.* 8 (1954), 128.

and J. A. Heady have examined the statistics of children of men in eight occupational groups and reported that the decline in both neo-natal and post-natal mortality was remarkably uniform between 1911 and 1950.[1]

The municipal ante-natal services are now used by all sections of the community. Whether supervision is afforded early enough is perhaps another matter. It would appear from the following table that those who were most likely to need early supervision were the last to come to the clinics.[2]

Percentage coming under supervision during each trimester of pregnancy by occupational group

	Wives of					
Percentage first attending during	Pro-fessional and salaried workers (%)	Black-coated wage earners (%)	Manual workers (%)	Agri-cultural workers (%)	Men in other occu-pations (%)	Un-married expectant mothers (%)
1st trimester	61·4	47·0	36·6	33·3	40·1	14·9
2nd trimester	27·7	39·4	45·6	47·8	40·5	38·0
3rd trimester	10·9	13·6	17·8	19·0	19·4	47·2
Total (%)	100·0	100·0	100·0	100·1	100·0	100·1

The same survey showed that in England and Wales thirty-two per cent of rural and forty-six per cent of urban confinements take place in hospital; but there are wide regional variations (p. 53). Three-quarters of the confinements of the professional and salaried workers take place in an institution (p. 55). This compares with the United States and Netherlands practice. Of White American babies eighty-one per cent were born in hospital and in some urban areas, for instance towns in Washington State, the percentage was ninety-nine. In Holland where home births are the objective of official policy eighty per cent take place at home, and the results, judged on the basis of the stillbirth rate and the maternal and neo-natal death rates, are most successful (p. 49).

[1] J. N. Morris and J. A. Heady, *Lancet* I (1955), 554.
[2] *Maternity in Great Britain.*

Of the women who were confined at home in Britain, thirty-two per cent were attended by doctors, and in a further four per cent the doctor is called in by the midwife. Sixty-four per cent of all home confinements were undertaken by midwives, of whom fifty-seven were municipal and seven per cent private (p. 65).

Attendances at the welfare centre tend to cease when the child begins to walk. Home visiting is then often the only method of health supervision, for it is probable that the doctor will be called in only if the child is acutely ill.

Criticism of child welfare services

The maternity and child welfare services have been the subject of a good deal of reassessment and some criticism. Perhaps the most comprehensive has been that of Professor A. Moncrieff,[1] of which the following seven points may be noticed:

(1) The welfare centres began, and largely continued, as a part of a campaign to reduce deaths in infancy from digestive disorders. They played an indirect part in the reduction of deficiency diseases, but the most valuable contributions to breast feeding management have been made by people outside this service such as Dr Harold Waller and Dr Charlotte Naish.

(2) Today, after the newborn period, it is the acute respiratory rather than the digestive disorders which present the major difficulties.

(3) There is not enough co-operation between the hospital, the G.P., and the child welfare services; this is especially serious in the case of premature babies. He refers to the report of the Biological and Medical Committee appointed by the Royal Commission on Population in 1950.

(4) J. E. Geddes (1950)[2] has stated that in Birmingham for the years 1946/49 the deaths under fifteen were as follows: scarlet fever, 2; diphtheria, 15; measles, 48; whooping cough, 114; T.B., 203; yet the tuberculin patch test is not always done in infant welfare centres.

(5) The epidemiology and pathogenesis of respiratory tract infections do not receive adequate attention from the centres, especially in the light of F. J. W. Miller's conclusion,[3] as a result of his work in Newcastle, that in the first five years of life acute infective disease is essentially a family infection.

[1] B.M.J. 2 (1950), 795. [2] Journal of the Royal Sanitary Institute, 70 (1950), 341.
[3] Public Health, 63 (1949), 61.

(6) Opportunities of establishing sound mental hygiene in the pre-school age-group are neglected. The percentage of 'psychological defects' are about the same as of otitis media and heart disease in the routine medical examinations in 1948 in the L.C.C. schools. The prevention of chronic ear trouble and of rheumatic heart disease is approached with more enthusiasm than is preventive mental hygiene.

(7) R. M. Dykes[1] has stated that, although Luton is a favoured town, infant mortality rates show a definite social gradient, whereas infant morbidity does not; the conclusion is that the lowering of infant death-rate will be achieved by ensuring that sick infants in the lower income groups get better and earlier attention. (More than half the total sickness in Luton was concentrated in less than seven per cent of the infants and those seven per cent were evenly distributed through the social classes. Incidence of illness increases with family size.)

Professor Moncrieff points out elsewhere that handicapped children are the responsibility of the school health service from the age of two and suggests that all pre-school children should be under the same service.[2]

Professor C. McNeil draws attention to the need to develop the somewhat neglected educational aspect of the services.[3] He is of the opinion that success in the promotion of health in childhood in the future rests with the child welfare services.

The curative work of the service in the treatment of many kinds of minor disorder and in the diagnosis of serious illness at the clinics is of great value. But more valuable is its preventive work. This has a double aim—(1) to reduce to a minimum the number of infant and child deaths, and (2) to raise to a maximum the quality of life in the survivors—and a single method of achieving it by the education of mothers in the manifold kinds of child care and in the right use of each...the first aim...has gone a long way towards achievement; the second...is only beginning.

He quotes John Burns who, when he was President of the Local Government Board, said: 'First concentrate on the mother. What the mother is the children are. The stream is no purer than the source. Let us glorify, dignify, purify motherhood by every means in our power.' To improve the educational aspect of the

---

[1] *Illness in Infancy* (Luton, 1950).
[2] *Child Health and the State* (Oxford, 1953), p. 11.   [3] *B.M.J.* 1 (1954), 533.

services it is important to have some factual information concerning mothers' difficulties. Breast-feeding, for example, seems to be declining. It appears that only about one-third of mothers are breast-feeding by the end of the third month, and that the rate, at this time, is higher in the upper than in the lower social classes. It is only very recently, however, that a study has been made of mothers feeding their babies within their own homes.[1] An intensive follow-up for three months was made of 106 primiparae who left Aberdeen Maternity Hospital breast-feeding. All but two of them experienced difficulty. Seventy-four abandoned it within three months. The most common complaints were of babies who cried excessively; maternal fatigue, breast and nipple complications, and inadequate lactation. Symptoms suggesting harm to the baby were more likely to result in weaning than were difficulties or discomforts affecting the mother only. The mothers who continued to lactate throughout the three months were more often unwell and worried than those who abandoned breast-feeding soon after leaving hospital, and the breast-fed baby had no obvious advantage. The investigators conclude, 'It seems that the breast-feeding mother in modern urban society often has to accept a heavy load of discomfort and disability, and that this is attributable more to her way of life than to the fact of breast-feeding *per se.*'

J. W. B. Douglas and J. M. Blomfield,[2] summing up their survey of a group of children drawn from all parts of Great Britain and from all social classes, kept under observation from birth, write (p. 141), 'The incidence and severity of both illness and accidents was more closely related to the standard of maternal care than to home conditions, and since there were large social group differences in the quality of maternal care we feel that this factor accounts for much of the excess of serious illness and death among the poorer children.' Their general conclusion is (p. 142): 'Indeed, it appears that the social and educational approach is still of primary importance in the saving of infant life.'

[1] F. E. Hytten, J. C. Yorston and A. M. Thomson, *B.M.J.* I (1958), 310.
[2] *Children Under Five* (London, 1958).

Health visitors

Practically every mother is visited by the health visitor within the first few weeks of life of her child, the medical officer of health having received the statutory notification of a birth in his area. The health visitors aim to provide the link between the family and the health service. They are now responsible for giving advice to the whole family, in their own homes, on the care of the sick and the spread of infection. (Formerly their supervision was confined to young children.) Their duties include the routine visiting of children, from birth to five years of age, to advise on their care and treatment. They also visit homes in connection with infectious diseases, particularly those affecting young children. They are in attendance at ante-natal and post-natal clinics, and they may also be concerned with the supervision of home helps and arrangements for the care of foster children whose maintenance is undertaken for reward. The local public health authority is responsible for the care and treatment of persons (including children) suffering from tuberculosis. Special visitors are appointed to supervise sufferers in their own homes, and to advise them on their specific health problems.

The health visitor is by qualification an S.R.N. who has her Part I midwifery examination and holds the certificate of her own institution. The Thousand Families survey criticised the present system of health visiting.[1] The child welfare service was ripe, it argued, for a reassessment of its work. Health visitors should be brought regularly into conference with the medical officer of health. 'The health visitor should, in her work, use her hands as well as her heart and mind. She should become a children's home nurse.'

Another inquiry took up the rather different point of the overlapping of welfare workers.[2] While the committee rejected the notion of a single general-purpose social worker for family visiting, they recommended the health visitor's close association with the general practitioner, who 'is tending to become the clinical leader

[1] *A Thousand Families in Newcastle upon Tyne* (1954), p. 182.
[2] *Inquiry into Health Visiting* (H.M.S.O. 1956), pp. viii, 110.

of the domiciliary health service team'. At the moment she probably visits on average one-quarter to two-fifths of the families in a doctor's practice: and if there were association rather than overlap, it would greatly add to the number of families whom she could visit. She might, also, relieve other workers of merely supportive visits. They also pointed out, too, that she could play 'an important, if unspectacular, role in relation to mental health. While their main importance may be in helping mothers, they should be able to take account of psychological factors in any case with which they deal.' As to this point, one difficulty may be noted: the health visitor rarely meets the child's father since her visits take place in normal working hours.

It is still too early to say how the services will develop, but it is fairly clear that the old separation of the maternity and child services and general practice are tending to disappear, and as doctors become more concerned with domiciliary conditions the benefit of a closer association with the health visitor is becoming apparent.

Maternity benefits

We have seen that the burden of children falls on couples when their earnings are rarely at a maximum, and the state makes provision for relieving part at least of the expense of children. The National Insurance scheme provides three maternity benefits—and where the conditions for each benefit are satisfied, all three may be paid for one confinement. A confinement is considered to have taken place not only when a living child is born, but, if pregnancy has lasted at least twenty-eight weeks, when a child is stillborn. The benefits are, first, the maternity grant, to help with the general expense of having a baby; second, the home confinement grant to help meet the extra expense when the baby is born elsewhere than in hospital accommodation provided at public cost; third, the maternity allowance, a weekly payment before and after confinement to women who ordinarily do paid work for an employer or on their own account. The allowance is intended to make it easier for them to give up work in good time before their confinement in the interests of themselves and their babies.

Furthermore, if it is not a first child, the mother is entitled to the family allowance of eight shillings for the second child and ten shillings for the third and each subsequent one.

SICK CHILDREN AT HOME

Various provisions are made for assisting the family where there is a sick child, one of them an old and respected service, and others experimental. The local authorities also may make provision.

District nurses are employed in most areas—formerly by local voluntary associations—to provide free or inexpensive nursing facilities within the home for families recommended by the doctor. Their function is, of course, not limited to nursing children. Most district nursing associations are ultimately affiliated to the Queen's Institute of District Nursing. In remote districts, the 'Queen's' nurse is often the general practitioner's mainstay.

Various experimental schemes have been evolved to assist the general practitioner in caring for the child sick at home or newly returned from hospital. Experiments carried out in Birmingham, Cardiff, Leeds and London, are particularly interesting.

Professor J. M. Smellie has reported that, as a result of the success of the Children's Nursing Unit established at Rotherham in 1949,[1] a similar service has been introduced in Birmingham

> to promote still further a live integration and close co-operation between general practitioner, local authority, and hospital service, the link being the district nurse... [to avoid] in-patient treatment in some cases, and in others [to achieve] discharge from hospital to home earlier than might otherwise be desirable. Thus, separation of the ill child from his mother and his home would be lessened, and possible psychological trauma minimised.[2]

All general practitioners practising in the selected area were told (*inter alia*) that nursing services would be available, on request, to assist them in the care and treatment of their sick child patients in their own homes. They would also have full and free access to any such child admitted to hospital. The plan was put into operation in

[1] See J. A. Gillet in *B.M.J.* I (1954), 684.   [2] *B.M.J.* I (1956), supp. 256.

October 1954 and in the first year 454 children had been visited in their homes. The principal diseases were respiratory infections, including 271 cases of tonsillitis and otitis; there were forty-four cases of abscesses and boils; thirty-one of skin conditions, and nineteen of infectious diseases. Twenty-six children required admission to hospital, including only two out of a total of nineteen cases of gastro-enteritis. In particular, evening visits have been found to be most effective in allaying the worries and anxieties of mothers, so that there have been very few emergency calls during the night.

In Cardiff two of the authority's health visitors have been seconded to work in hospitals.[1] Their duties are divided between hospital attendances and home visiting. They attend ward rounds and contribute to the medico-social histories of the children concerned. By visits to the homes they help to prepare the parents for the return of the child and in co-operation with the family doctor and the local health visitor they continue to visit the child after its discharge, ensuring its attendance at follow-up clinics, and giving advice on various problems.

In Leeds there is a similar scheme for midwives.[2] Particular attention is paid to the difficulties of mothers whose babies have been detained in hospital because of illness and prematurity and who are suddenly confronted with the difficulties of feeding when the baby is discharged.

In London in April 1954 a mobile team of two paediatricians, a sister, two nurses and a part-time physiotherapist was formed at St Mary's Hospital.[3] The system of home care has a special place in the treatment of medical conditions where education in preventive methods is important: feeding difficulties and gastro-enteritis, for example, and in the treatment of children who are under five or have chronic or incurable disease. The London experimenters believe that nearly a quarter of the children in hospital during a

[1] A. G. Watkins in B.M.J. I (1951), 1075.
[2] W. S. Craig, G. A. Kitching, I. G. Davies and C. Fraser Brockington in B.M.J. I (1951), 1234.
[3] R. Lightwood, F. S. W. Brimblecombe, J. D. L. Reinhold, E. D. Burnard and J. A. Davis in Lancet, I (1957), 313.

review period were admitted for conditions which could have been managed at home, if the doctors had possessed the facilities and experience required, and that there were other children whose stay in hospital could have been shortened. They emphasise that in hospital responsibility for the patient passes into the hands of the hospital staff, and decisions that could affect the child's whole future may be taken without reference to the family doctor, who is normally the person best able to relate an illness to the social context. 'Such a reduction in the influence and responsibility of the family doctor is not in the patient's interests, especially in paediatrics, where symptoms are often pointers to a strain involving the whole family.'

The Ministry of Health recommended in 1944 that local authorities provide for the domiciliary care of premature infants. Many do provide for the attendance of midwives or health visitors capable of teaching mothers the special care required when the medical practitioner decides that the infant is to be nursed at home. Provision for the loan of equipment is made—special cots, clothing, hot-water bottles, feeding bottles and mucus extractors. Milk banks for premature infants may be established and maintained either by hospitals or local authorities. The local authority has a duty to provide a home nursing service and may provide home helps.

CHAPTER IX

THE CHILD AT SCHOOL

When children are first grouped together, be it in the day nursery or at school, it is not long before the consequences of the aggregation bring them to the doctor. Before schooling begins, most children have for shorter or longer periods been in contact with children and adults who are not within the immediate circle. At the nursery or school, however, the child embarks upon membership of a new, long-continuing and more or less stable group. In doing so, he is faced with the need to make new adaptations, and it is for this reason that the doctor's help is often required. The problems may be physical demands or they may be mental—exposure to new axioms, self-evident assumptions and beliefs, and the ways of conduct erected upon them, which differ from those of his home.

PRE-SCHOOL FACILITIES

Parents are required by the Education Acts to provide their children over five years of age with an education. Some children begin school in nursery classes at three; others begin in a nursery school at two and some experience group care in a day nursery at any time from the age of one month.

Day nurseries

The nursery school and day nursery are different in their aims. The day nursery is primarily interested in the children's health; if it is a public one, it is administered by the maternity and child welfare authority, and a trained nurse is in charge. Children may be received from the age of one month but cannot be kept beyond school age. The nursery provides for children throughout the industrial day, week and year.

There was a very considerable growth of day nurseries during the war, for the argument was that the infant of a woman skilled, for example, in aircraft work, could be looked after in the day nursery, so that his mother could return to production quickly. But the nurseries are expensive to maintain and their value to the children has been debated. M. E. McLaughlin has reported on the entire population of eight Ministry of Health wartime day nurseries in Birmingham in 1944–5, and compared them with eight control groups of children at home in the neighbourhoods of the nurseries.[1] The nursery children received their meals without the surrender of coupons and they could thus have almost twice as much food as the children at home. Yet for all age groups, both boys and girls, the proportion of children brought up at home whose general condition was classified as 'good' or 'very good' was significantly higher than that of nursery children.

The nursery children had a significantly higher incidence of tonsillar enlargement, of enlarged cervical glands, of chronic nasopharyngeal infection and of the physical signs of bronchitis. Subacute and acute nasopharyngeal infections were significantly higher for nursery boys but not above chance for nursery girls.

McLaughlin (p. 631) also found that the nursery children under two years were lighter than home children but that those over two years were heavier—the differences for girls over two were not significant. The total incidence of varicella, mumps and pertussis was small but measles in epidemic form was present during the investigation and the incidence was markedly heavier in the nurseries, especially among the younger ones. Signs of fatigue were noted in the nursery group: there was, for example, a higher incidence of *pes valgus*, which may be associated with the long hours kept by the nursery children. Similar results were obtained from a survey of 4587 children examined in twenty-two local government areas in Great Britain.[2]

The general practice is for an assistant medical officer of health to carry out a routine medical inspection at monthly intervals. The

[1] *B.M.J.* 1 (1947), 591.
[2] Medical Women's Federation in *B.M.J.* 2 (1946), 217.

medical officer keeps an eye on all health matters in the nurseries pertaining to the welfare of the children. All children are medically examined on admission. The children are received daily by the matron or deputy matron, and any child thought to be suffering from an infectious disease is excluded or isolated until seen by the doctor.

Nursery schools

The nursery schools are primarily interested in the children's social education, and they are run sometimes voluntarily, sometimes as private schools, sometimes by the local education authority; they are in the charge of a certificated teacher. Children are rarely received under two and may attend in some until they are seven. The school has a short school day and the ordinary school week, term and year.

The two- or three-year-old, it is assumed, is ready to associate with other children. He is mobile, has a vocabulary that enables him to deal with simple social situations and is also more or less house-trained. Middle-class parents often experience real difficulty in finding other children for their own to play with. This problem is essentially a middle-class one. In a working-class neighbourhood, with smaller dwellings closer together and a slightly higher fertility, there are nearly always other children to play with. The working-class toddler is much more likely to be in need of safe playing space than of companionship. As households become smaller, the importance of the nursery school, as a means of relieving the single-handed mother of the growing demands of her toddlers, especially when another child is on the way, increases.

PRIMARY SCHOOLS

The parents' duty is to provide their children with an education and there is some freedom allowed them in doing so. The local education authority is informed of the births in its area and has a duty to provide a place of education for every child. If it appears to the local education authority that the parents are failing in their duty, the authority must serve a notice on the parent requiring him to satisfy the authority to the contrary within fourteen days. The official of the education authority directly concerned was formerly called the attendance officer. Today he is referred to as the welfare officer. If the parents fail, an attendance order is served, after a further fourteen days' notice, to attend a school named in the order. The only defence is that the child is receiving full-time education elsewhere, suitable to his age, ability and aptitude.

Parents may be summoned for failing to send their children to school regularly. The parent may successfully plead that the child was sick or unavoidably prevented, that the day of absence was one of religious observance or that the school is not within walking distance (two miles for children under eight; three miles for others) and the local authority has provided neither transport nor boarding accommodation. Even so, it is not easy to get canal children, fair-children, 'travellers', or gypsy children to school: they slip in and out of the educational net as they move with their parents, as indeed do the children of the better-off whose parents, from occupation or inclination, are constantly on the move. Children must be sent to school as regularly as the trade or employment of the parents permit, but attendance must not fall below 200 times in twelve months.

Some freedom is allowed for choice among the local authority schools. Parents need not send their children to the nearest school. They may, for example, choose a school of their own religious persuasion, or, if this is impracticable, may withdraw their child from class when religious instruction of which they disapprove is given. The education authority must provide the place, however, and if access can be obtained only by, say, boat or taxi, they must, whatever the expense, provide the boat or taxi. They may in due course prudently decide that a child in an isolated home should be given residential education. It is but very rarely that the parents can provide the succession of teachers and tutors necessary for an education today. Practically every normal child is bound to submit to schooling. It need not, of course, be schooling provided by the local authority.

Where the local authority is satisfied that a child cannot obtain the education suited to his ability and aptitude except by attendance at a direct grant or independent school, the authority may be expected to meet the full boarding fees. For children whose attendance at direct grant or independent boarding schools is considered desirable by the parents and is approved by the local authority, a partial or total contribution towards fees and boarding expenses may be allowed, the income of the parents being taken into consideration. The lack of a school of a particular religious denomination within daily travelling distance is not of itself considered a sufficient ground for provision of boarding education.

Service education grants are available for those parents in the services who find it necessary to send children aged over eleven to a boarding school in the United Kingdom or to board them out with a relative or friend so that they may continue to attend a particular day school. The grant is limited to service parents who although for the time being in the United Kingdom are normally unlikely to remain in their present place of duty for more than four years. These grants are not in substitution of other assistance but are an addition to income.

Employment of school children

Children should remain at school until the end of the term in which they attain their fifteenth birthday. In fact some children work before that, especially in agricultural districts. In Scotland it is still necessary to exempt children from attendance at school to assist in lifting the potato crop if the acreage devoted to this vital crop is not to be drastically curtailed.[1] The production of mechanical harvesters able to work efficiently under Scottish conditions is the only feasible alternative in the immediately foreseeable future under conditions of full employment. London children for generations have disappeared from school just after term has begun after the summer holidays to accompany their parents to the hop-fields.

No child who is more than two years below the upper limit of compulsory school age may be employed before 6.0 a.m. or after 8.0 p.m. on any day or for more than two hours on a school day

[1] *Employment of Children in the Potato Harvest* (H.M.S.O. 1956).

or on a Sunday; he may not lift, carry or move anything so heavy as to be likely to cause injury to him. Local authorities may make bye-laws authorising employment of children by parents or guardians in light agricultural or horticultural work, prohibiting employment in specified industries, prescribing conditions of employment. Children under sixteen are prohibited from street trading except when employed by their parents. Children over twelve may be licensed by the local education authority of the area to take part in any specified entertainment provided the authority is satisfied that the child is fit, is kindly treated and that arrangements have been made for his education.

The Ministry of Education

During their primary schooling children are early 'streamed'. Schools may be expected to have three streams: 'A' stream, the brighter, 'B' the middling and 'C' the duller children. The three streams will go at different paces and will use suitably different methods according to the ability of the children.

What is taught in the schools is not prescribed in detail. The Ministry of Education offers general observations concerning the curriculum and a good deal of advice; but the duty of running the schools falls on the local education authority.

The Ministry has its own inspectors who are concerned with the efficiency of the school. They are also anxious to give the benefit of their advice and experience. The Ministry's control is essentially through the purse: the financing of education cannot be done entirely locally and it is in the giving or withholding of grants and the conditions upon which the grants are made that the control of the Ministry is primarily maintained.

The submission of detailed estimates of proposed expenditure and detailed and explicit conditions laid down by the Ministry for the making of its grants, together with the right to inspect, give the sort of central control to education without abolishing either the individual authority's responsibility in law or its degree of freedom, both of which are general in British administration. The Government is proposing to change the system with effect from April

1959.[1] They propose to make 'block grants' to local authorities. 'The Government must then remain responsible for laying down national policy and for ensuring compliance with basic standards in the revised services which are aided by grants. Controls for this purpose will be limited to the "key points" of a service—though for this maximum local discretion will be given in the method of providing the service: the reward of efficiency will accrue wholly to the benefit of the local population.' There is some apprehension that some local authorities may be tempted to economise on education.

The local authority

The local authority—county or county borough—appoints a number of elected councillors to form the education committee. They are not experts on education, merely ordinary men and women to whom has been delegated the local public responsibility to provide education as directed by Parliament in the Education Acts. Answerable to them is an administrative staff, whose chief officer is generally called the Director of Education. School staffs have professional educational qualifications, and it is the responsibility of the headmaster or mistress to draw up the detailed syllabus for his or her school. The local authority appoints inspectors who see that the policy of the education committee is carried out within the schools.

Schools maintained by a local education authority are either those provided by the authority itself or by 'voluntary' bodies, usually one of the religious denominations, where the authority shares responsibility. Each voluntary school has its board of managers or governors. In the 'controlled' school, the managers, two-thirds of whom are appointees of the local education authority, must be consulted on the appointment of the head teacher and of any teacher who will give denominational instruction. In the 'aided' school, the managers are responsible for the exterior of the building and all improvements, enlargements and alterations, half the cost of which may be reimbursed by the Minister. They appoint the staff and control religious instruction. One-third of the managers

[1] *Local Government Finance* (H.M.S.O. 1957).

are local authority appointees. 'Special agreement' schools are those few schools which had begun to develop before the war along the lines permitted by the Education Act 1936 and ran into difficulties—because, for example, they were actually rebuilding, bound by a contract, and unable to continue—when the war broke out.

Some Local Education Authority problems

All local education authorities have faced enormous problems since the war. The whole of the complicated and laboriously built system of education, the subject of constant criticism and the victim of many economies, was turned upside down by the events of the war. Under-staffed, with some damaged and many obsolete buildings, the education authorities found themselves in 1944 called upon to provide sound and comprehensive educational services, planned in three stages; for primary, secondary and further education, and the difficulties are by no means over today.

(1) *Buildings*

The quality of school buildings provided by the local education authority varies enormously. In new areas the schools may well be new and incorporate the latest refinements. In the older districts schools are nearly always out of date. Many were built to provide for the children coming into the schools in the 1870's and have been black-listed by the Ministry for years. One or two were rebuilt before the war, and where an occasional school was destroyed in the war a modern building has been erected, but in the old areas with declining populations the prospect of providing schools adequate by modern standards is remote.

R. McKinnon Wood, a past chairman of the London County Council Education Committee, is reported to have said that the housing shortage in East London was such that no sites were as yet available for school buildings. With 60,000 people in the first category of priority on the waiting list, the authorities were forced to reserve all suitable sites for slum clearance. If the plans for educational buildings were carried out without delay, over 300,000 people would have to surrender their homes.[1]

[1] *Times Educational Supplement*, 23 November 1956.

Many rural schools are badly equipped.[1] One hundred and thirty-four replies were received to an unspecified number of questionnaires sent to three (unidentified) widely separated rural areas of England. One in three had bucket or earth-closet sanitation, some unusable in winter. One in eight relied for water on wells which usually dry up in summer. Two in seven have a hot-water supply, but a further two in seven obtain their hot water only from the school canteen. One in ten is lighted by oil lamps.

(2) Staff

The ratio in the nursery school is roughly one member of staff to five children: in the better preparatory and private schools it is somewhere between one member of staff to ten or twelve pupils. Although few public-school masters have a professional diploma to teach, the great majority are equipped with an upper second or first-class degree. The 1944 Ministry of Education Regulation (after the Butler Act that prescribed, among other things, secondary education for all children), recommended that the number of children per class should be forty in the primary schools and thirty in secondary schools. In Birmingham over half the primary schools and nearly half the secondary schools have classes of between forty-one and fifty children. It may appear curious to those who emphasise the individual needs of the younger child that the number recommended per class should be greater in their case. For those who value instruction, however, it seems obvious that the older children call for more individual teaching.

There are local difficulties in recruiting teachers. The poorer districts—Walsall, Birmingham, Hull, metropolitan Essex—are particularly badly off. Some authorities have an unaccountably large 'turn-over' of staff. The Ministry of Education is asking the authorities with higher staff ratios to limit their recruiting. It is possible that after 1960, when the immediately post-war children who create 'the bulge' have passed through the schools, there will be enough teachers to increase the ratio of teachers to children generally and, if recruitment is maintained, to establish a three-year (instead

[1] *Head Teachers' Review*, 48 (November 1957), 169.

of two-year) teacher-training course. There was an agreed and publicly expressed hope, during the period of reconstruction, that children would remain at school until they were sixteen. The shortage of teachers and of buildings makes this impossible and the age when schooling may finish remains at fifteen.

Salaries are low in comparison with professional scales except in the public schools, and, with this reservation again, the ladder of advancement is short and undistinguished. The social status of the schoolmaster is in consequence not very high—not that this is a characteristic peculiar to Britain. One of the few real exceptions is among Orthodox Jews. Here 'learning' is essentially a masculine pursuit. The male teachers of the very young are not the highly skilled but those who failed to climb the ladder: the ladder is very much present, however, and those who climb are very highly regarded. Orthodox Jewish women do not so much teach their children as care for them. On the other hand in the West generally, and perhaps to a greater extent in North America, teaching both at home and at school, has become essentially the women's job.

Very serious shortages have arisen generally because science graduates are attracted into industry at salaries considerably greater than education authorities can pay. Particular difficulties arise in poor and industrial areas where accommodation is in short supply and where teachers in demand elsewhere are reluctant to go. The shortage is critical in Birmingham, for example, and the mal-distribution of teachers is a major problem. A leader in *The Times Educational Supplement* (14 September 1956) says: '... whereas some areas like Wales are satiated with teachers, so that they can be retired as soon as may be and the married women are dismissed to fret at home, other places like Birmingham and the Midlands generally are desperate for the want of them now, and as the rolls mount may find their school systems threatened with breakdown.'

(3) *Intake*

Children do not flow through schools regularly: national events cause the birth-rate to fluctuate and cause general difficulty: bad years like 1935 are unfruitful years; so, too, are war years; the first years of peace are fruitful. The offspring of the couples reunited after the war are well on their way through the schools and will soon be entering the universities. Local authorities have their peculiar difficulties: a new housing estate where the couples are young will have many school entrants and few senior children. In time the schools will be full and the parents nearing the end of their reproductive period, but still occupying their houses: the school population will then fall off at the lower end. In the meantime the young adults, if they are to have homes of their own, will move away and multiply elsewhere.

SECONDARY SCHOOLS

'The eleven plus'

The Education Act prescribes that at the age of eleven children should be selected by aptitude and ability to benefit by the most suitable form of education. There has been considerable argument about the methods of this selection. Even before the Act, the traditional written examination had been falling in esteem for these children because of their youth, because results reflected the efficiency of teaching and not necessarily native ability, and because children might be coached solely for the examination to the detriment of their general education. A single measure was needed which would classify children by native ability—and so the system of selection by intelligence test was introduced. The object was to detect those children who would be good with their heads and should go to grammar schools and those who would be good with their hands and should go to technical schools, and to provide a new kind of school—the secondary modern—for the rest. It is important that it be remembered that the object was to be absolutely fair to the child: if an inexact analogy may be used, they were, like cars, to be classified by a simply ascertainable measure of horsepower and not by the skill of the driver in racing the car, by the hard work of the mechanics in getting it ready, or by its gadgets.[1]

[1] A review of the relevant information concerning the tests may be found by P. E. Vernon (ed.), *Secondary School Selection* (London, 1957).

Criticism of the tests grew apace. First it was suspected, then demonstrated and then admitted, that children did better on the tests if coached; and the view not unnaturally grew that it would be better if all children were coached, since the maximum effect of coaching is soon achieved. Secondly, doubt grew as to what the tests measured. The current moderate view is that between one-half and three-quarters of the attributes measured are closely associated with genetic endowment. An interesting criticism of a basic assumption for this view has been put forward: that there is no proof that native ability is randomly distributed about the normal Gaussian curve. The argument says that if it appears to be so, this is because of the distribution of the inequalities of environment upon something evenly distributed. This is to argue that all men are born equal. Watson and the Behaviourists argued it: many devoted teachers in poor areas believe in it. Today the notion that all except the obviously handicapped are equally endowed is a Russian concept: it finds support among British communists;[1] but in the West it is held to be contrary to common observation and to the concepts of biology and physiology. The egalitarian case is put by Brian Simon.[2]

Thirdly, it was suspected that whether the factor was genetic or not, the tests were merely grading children according to their ability to do the work of schools which had high social approval—the grammar schools: some may value that sort of ability, particularly the traditionalists and many parents, but that of itself does not establish that the selected children have 'more' of anything—except the ability to do scholastic work.

Fourthly, assuming that what was tested was the capacity, or ability, to learn anything, it was asked why all the greater ability should be creamed away from technical education, especially at a time when the growing need was for great technical expansion.

Practical difficulties arise, too. Whatever the tests may show, the education of a child at eleven plus (or any other age for that matter)

[1] *Times Educational Supplement*, 27 October 1950.
[2] *Intelligence Testing and the Comprehensive School* (London, 1954). A critique of the mathematical concepts can be found in D. G. Lewis, *Brit. J. Psychol.* **48** (1957), 98. Sir Cyril Burt (*ibid.* p. 161) has replied.

is governed in part by the type of education available. Some local authorities have no provision for technical education, and very few can take more than fifteen per cent of the eleven plus children for technical education. Grammar-school provision is even more un-even: Merionethshire has two-thirds of its eleven plus children in grammar schools whereas many authorities can provide for but ten per cent. A growing minority of authorities has abandoned the tests and some, including the largest, combine the tests with teachers' assessments.

As the demand increases for more technicians, more technical education, more places must be found. Possibly as greater efficiency penetrates into administration and offices become more mechan-ised, fewer purely administrative jobs may be available and the social differences and the concept of education based upon the ideal of a white-collar career may blur if not disappear.

During the earlier years of school the education authority is dis-covering, and providing special facilities for, subnormal children, whether their handicap is mental or physical. The classification at eleven plus is concerned with detecting the mentally superior child. Very little attention is given to those who have some physical superiority, such as ability in sports or dancing. It is not impossible for a child to become a ballet dancer at the expense of the local education authority, or a painter, or a musician: but the athlete in Britain is still, largely, a self-made man and relatively little atten-tion is given to physical education.

Doris Baker, writing of the medical examination of women in the Army Recruit Training Centres, says, 'The result, so far as the women were concerned, revealed a gross degree of physical indiscipline and, more striking still, a complete lack of pride of body and appreciation of physical fitness.'[1] She draws attention, too, to a fact that is regularly avoided in educational writing: 'There will always be a certain number of children whose intellect will never be of the first order, who will have to earn their living by

---

[1] D. M. Baker, 'Physical Education and the Health of the Child' in A. Mon-crieff and W. A. R. Thomson (eds.), *Child Health* (Practitioner Handbooks, London, 1952), p. 189.

manual work, and rely on their muscles rather than their minds. For these children, physical fitness is an even greater necessity; it is the nation's duty to do everything possible to develop the physically immature.' J. N. Oliver has shown that with systematic physical conditioning a small group of Birmingham educationally subnormal boys improved in their attitude to life because of their improved health and vitality.[1]

The comprehensive school

In a nation containing many ways of life, with religious tolerance and a range of political belief, education which is publicly provided is perhaps bound to be the subject of controversy. Recently the differences of opinion have centred around the comprehensive school. The case for these schools was based upon the advantages of large numbers, which make possible otherwise unattainable equipment and services and give opportunities for the fine grading of children within a wide range of subjects taught with the possibility of regarding and streaming misplaced children. By means of having grammar, technical and modern courses under one roof or on one site it was hoped to create new loyalties and obliterate social differences, and incidentally avoid the inevitable social problems which arise in a family when the children are allocated to different schools, or when a working-class father has a son at the middle-class grammar school. The case for the retention, with improvements, of the old schools rested upon the small numbers of pupils at each, which made possible an otherwise unattainable personal contact between child and staff and particularly between the child and the head of the school, and which gave the child the opportunity of sharing in a long tradition and of identifying himself with a valued way of life deeply rooted in the past.

In practice convenience has dictated the choice of comprehensive schools in some areas, Anglesey and the Isle of Man, for example, while in others, London, for example, they have been built by the local authorities, so far as they have been permitted, in pursuit of their ideas.

[1] In *Med. Off.* **97** (1957), 19.

There has been speculation and willingness to experiment. Croydon has canvassed the idea of bringing together all sixth forms to form a 'junior college', but the plan was never executed. R. Pedley has put forward a plan for comprehensive schools of about five hundred pupils for all children under fifteen and thereafter a high school which some would attend part-time, others full-time, for three years.[1] Both these plans aim to give the feeling of adult status to senior boys which is lacking in town and day grammar schools.

W. P. Alexander, the Secretary of the Association of Education Committees, suggests providing for the five per cent of super-normal children in special high schools in a way similar to the provision for the handicapped. One very practical reason which he puts forward is that 5000 secondary schools have an average intake of only 370 pupils. To replace these schools would take ten to fifteen years and cost some £700 million.[2]

The Leicestershire Education Committee embarked in September 1957 on an experiment whereby there is no eleven-plus examination, but all children transfer at eleven to high schools except the bright ones who do so at ten. The high schools are the present secondary modern ones. At fourteen pupils may transfer, without examination, to the grammar school, provided that their parents undertake to keep them there until sixteen years.[3]

The secondary modern school

Currently the need is felt to re-orientate the educational system to the inevitable demands of the new technical revolution; but the great challenge to education of the past decade or so has been the establishment of the secondary modern school. Somehow, in the same old buildings, with much the same staff, something more than 'the extra year' has been introduced: there has been born the desire to educate the boy and girl who showed no inclination for,

---

[1] *Comprehensive Education* (London, 1956).
[2] *Times Educational Supplement*, 7 December 1956.
[3] *Ibid.* 12 April 1957.

or ability in, school subjects. It is perhaps as well to recall the words of that not unintellectual churchman, William Temple, when he was advocating the raising of the school-leaving age:

> The main ground is the necessity of providing a social life or community in which the individual may feel that he has a real share and for which he may feel a genuine responsibility....He needs a society of people about his own age, in the activities of which he may take a share equal to that of any other member, so that it may reasonably claim his loyalty, and he may have the sense of being wanted in it. Nothing else will draw out from him the latent possibilities of his nature.[1]

Left without the County Colleges, which were designed for part-time education after the age of sixteen, with the 'day-release' scheme for boys and girls in industry spreading but slowly and with the school-leaving age raised only to fifteen and not to sixteen, the modern schools might well have settled merely to the extra year. On the whole, this has not been so. Local authorities have built where they could, as imaginative new secondary modern as new grammar or comprehensive schools. Some teachers have felt spurred to bring their secondary modern school as far along the grammar-school path as personal enthusiasm and ingenuity will permit: in a written reply by the Parliamentary Secretary, the Ministry of Education has stated that in England and Wales in 1956 nearly 9000 secondary modern school pupils entered for the General Certificate of Education, and were successful in about half the subjects for which they entered.[2] Other teachers have genuinely sought to develop secondary modern schools along their own lines. Edward Blishen said in the course of a broadcast:

> For better or worse, we worry now in the secondary modern school at the problem of providing a certain amount of common ground between our two nations. We are not happy that there should still be hostility and acute misunderstanding when, in the persons of the young teacher and the secondary modern child, the two nations meet....The unhappy secondary modern school today is likely to be that which has clung to the old, shut-in, near-medieval classroom con-

---

[1] A. E. Baker, *William Temple and his Message* (London, 1946), p. 228.
[2] *Observer*, 24 February 1957.

THE CHILD AT SCHOOL

vention, while the happy one is the school that is bursting out of its class-rooms....School is a place to which one comes to learn about life and to consider it and to acquire ways of dealing with it: but it must not be a place that is in any way sealed off from life.[1]

It may well be that the Ministry of Education spokesman was right in his explanation for the fact that nearly 250,000 of the half-million children who could be expected to compete for the 100,000 grammar-school places each year were not doing so. Having pointed out that some children would be ruled out by preliminary tests, he said 'They [parents] are being guided by two things: the advice of the children's teachers; and the realisation that a grammar school is not the best type of school for every child.' Acceptance of this is, however, largely dependent upon the parents' realisation that the secondary modern school can have something to offer.

There has been a good deal of uneasiness felt about the general standard of local authority schools in basic subjects. Just after the War, reading ability among one per cent of school-leavers was, in comprehension, as low as that of the average seven-year-old in the schools in 1938 and thirty per cent had a 'reading age' less than that of twelve years on 1938 standards.[2] Among adults it was estimated that some seventeen per cent never rose above this standard. Whereas it was estimated that during the war standards had fallen away by 12 months and 22 months for pupils of eleven and fifteen respectively, by 1956 there had been an improvement on 1948 standards of 9 months by eleven-year-olds and 5 months by fifteen-year-olds.[3]

As important as attainment in the basic subjects is the attitude of the children. Some from 'better' homes undoubtedly feel a sense of failure because they did not secure a grammar-school 'place' at the eleven plus examination. A great many of them, however, are looking forward to taking their place in the world and are envious of their friends at work with their new independence and money.

[1] *Listener*, 21 February 1957.
[2] *Reading Ability*, Ministry of Education Pamphlet, no. 18 (H.M.S.O. 1950).
[3] *Standards of Reading, 1948–1956*, Ministry of Education Pamphlet no. 32 (H.M.S.O. 1957).

Schools do not find this anticipation easy to harness for educational purposes: the children are felt to be critical of the values of the school and challenge the staff on subjects which the staff may wish to avoid. Educationalists are not always prepared to accept the world as it is, and to take over mental-health notions of 'adjustment': of preparing children merely for the reality of the bus, the bench, the dogs, the wage-packet and the week-end. Growing children must be expected to be critical. The problem is how to turn their attitude towards the educationalists' ideals. The schools are vulnerable concerning the subjects which they may wish to avoid, and of these sex is of growing and engrossing interest to the secondary modern child. It is a sober fact that the single female school-mistress is on many counts at a disadvantage in the eyes of her fifteen-year-olds.

The secondary modern girls will never have the training in domestic service which came the way of so many of their grandmothers who were employed as domestics in middle-class households. The problem of how to educate them as lovers, wives and mothers remains largely unspoken of and unresolved. Whether the quietly flourishing 'finishers' for the older middle-class girls of the post-war period—probably of not much more than secondary modern ability—will provide a model, remains to be seen.

The median age for marriage has fallen since the war—and girls remain longer at school now. Both boys and girls grow heavier and taller faster than hitherto and 'as in the case of growth, comparison of early and recent British studies strongly suggests that sexual maturation is occurring significantly earlier at the present time than 50 years ago'.[1] The fact that schoolgirls are sexually interested may be masked in the technical or grammar schools: it must be faced in the secondary modern. In the grammar and technical schools a good deal of wastage may be attributed to the failure to understand the girls' outlook. M. Gallagher, in order to ascertain how far the prospect of marriage does deter secondary

[1] R. W. B. Ellis, 'Puberty and Adolescence', in R. W. B. Ellis (ed.), *Child Health and Development* (London, 1956), p. 208.

grammar and secondary technical school girls from continuing their education at school and afterwards, questioned 190 girls among those who left school between July 1947 and July 1950 in Wallasey, a residential district in the industrial and commercial area of Merseyside.[1] He found that seventy-four per cent left school earlier than the sixth form; that less than half undertook occupations which embodied further education; that of the sixty-seven per cent who were vocationally ambitious only twenty-two per cent had undertaken constructive measures to further their ambitions: that three-quarters intended to give up their work on marriage; that nearly half became married or engaged during the six years after leaving school. His general conclusion was that the prospect of marriage appeared to hinder many girls from undertaking further education, that their abilities were not fully developed and that an expensive form of education was often largely wasted. He stated that further research was needed into the question of how best the adolescent girl's interest in further education can be encouraged, with particular emphasis on the differentiation of the curriculum for boys and girls.

OTHER SCHOOLS

(1) *Direct grant*

Not all schools are under the control of the local authority. Some 200 receive a grant direct from the Ministry of Education. These schools are for fee-paying pupils and nearly all are grammar schools. In return for their grant they must offer twenty-five per cent of 'free places': places free to pupils who have previously attended for at least two years grant-aided primary schools. These are normally offered to the local education authority, which pays the fees. A further twenty-five per cent are 'reserved places' which the local authority may take up but not necessarily for children from grant-aided primary schools.

[1] M. Gallagher, *Brit. J. Educ. Psychol.* **27** (1957), 24.

(2) *Independent*

In England and Wales there are a further 5000 independent schools ranging from the great public school to those teaching a mere handful of children. All these schools are open to inspection by her Majesty's Inspectors and about one quarter of them are 'recognised as efficient'. The application for recognition is entirely at the discretion of the school.

(3) *Assisted*

An 'assisted' school is one to whose proprietors the local authority makes a grant, or makes payments for educational facilities provided, for example, for pupils nominated by it.

Part III of the Education Act 1944 provided for the establishment of a register of independent schools and it is now illegal to run a school not registered or provisionally registered. It will now be possible to compel the closure of unsuitable schools and the disqualification of unsuitable teachers.

MEDICAL PROVISION FOR SCHOOLS

Children are received into school at the beginning of the term after their fifth birthday. In the rest of Europe children start school later, and in British schools formal education does not usually begin immediately at five; some advocate that it should be delayed until about seven. The full school day is long for the five-year-old and occasionally, though not effectively, the suggestion is made, sometimes in connection with the want of school buildings, of raising the age of entry of children or restricting them to half-day school while they are small.

Problems are often presented to the family doctor which arise directly out of the stresses and strains of early school life, and the education authorities are themselves on the look-out for them, not only in normal children but also in those who for mental or physical reasons should receive special education. In the early years, too, the authorities will exclude some children as ineducable.

The local authority is required to provide for the medical inspection of all children in schools maintained by them. It is required to make arrangements for free medical treatment, and to encourage and assist children to make use of it. Both the general practitioner and the school medical officer have, therefore, a responsibility to the school-age child. Arrangements have grown up for the interchange of reports and discussion between them before a child is referred for specialist treatment, and hospital boards arrange for the same information to be passed to both upon the discharge of patients of school age. Some education authorities engage general practitioners, part-time, for inspection sessions. Children are examined by the school doctor sometime at the beginning, middle and end of their school career, and also as often as may be required to supervise the progress of any remedial treatment which has been recommended. Children in special schools are routinely examined once a year. The examination takes place in the school and there is consultation with the teaching staff; except in residential schools, parents are invited to be present. Children may also be seen at any inspection at the suggestion of the head teacher or, in London, the Care Committee. Private schools may have arrangements with the local authority to be included in the scheme. Children are seen once a term by a nurse, when the main purpose is to investigate personal hygiene. The nurse is present at the doctor's inspection and at the examination clinics, and carries out the work of the treatment centre. She examines the children for defects of vision and hearing and may give health instruction and home follow-up visits. Children found to be infested with vermin are sent to the cleansing station provided by the local public health authority to undergo the necessary treatment and to have their clothing disinfested. Special dental inspections are arranged periodically. Before 1944 there was no obligation on the part of the parent to submit the child to examination; since that date, however, it has been compulsory.

Medical and dental treatment may be obtained for school children in three ways: through the Health Service or private doctor; through the local authority school treatment centres, which provide, ordinarily, for minor ailments, defects of teeth, vision, speech and nutrition, and also, for example, for ringworm, rheumatism and enuresis; and through the hospitals by appointment. The larger education authorities appoint treatment organisers who attend hospitals to channel in children.

Special provision for handicapped children

The local education authority is required to make special provision for the education of children suffering from physical or mental disabilities and to provide special schools, where possible, for the seriously handicapped. Education continues until sixteen and must be begun as early as possible—sometimes from the age of two.

During the first year or so of schooling the local education authority will have classified the children who are subnormal, either mentally or physically, and made special provision for them. It will also have rejected some children as ineducable in a school.

The following estimates are made by the Ministry of Education:

Approximated expected frequencies of the main handicaps per 1000 registered pupils[1]

Blind	0·2–0·3
Partially sighted	1·0
Deaf	0·7–1·0
Partially deaf	1·0+
Delicate	1–2 per cent
Diabetic	No estimate available
Epileptic	0·2
Educationally subnormal	10 per cent
Maladjusted	About 1 per cent
Physically handicapped	5–8
Speech defects	1·5–3 per cent

Social factors in classification

The estimates for the educationally subnormal stand out from the rest as being of a different order. Ten per cent of children, the Ministry estimates, will manage their school work so poorly that they will need special education wholly or in part in substitution

[1] Adapted from *Special Educational Treatment*, Ministry of Education Pamphlet No. 5 (H.M.S.O. 1946).

for the education normally given in ordinary schools. This is obtained either by special teaching in 'backward' (or, as some prefer, 'opportunity') classes or in special E.S.N. schools—these latter the Ministry recommends should be provided for one per cent of the school population. This proportion few authorities achieve.[1] It is a matter of comment that the Ministry estimates that between five and ten times as many children will be educationally subnormal as will be physically delicate. The estimates show that children are being prepared for a civilisation which requires a general standard of mental activity so high that ten per cent of children are unlikely to achieve it. The physical demands, however, are not so heavy—any child can sit on a chair and push a pen—and as far as these are concerned, an anxious speculative eye need be turned on a much smaller percentage of children. The percentage of children labelled educationally subnormal is in part at least a measure of the society within which a child finds itself.

More than that: within the British Isles the labelling in practice, may well be a measure of the local educational standards rather than something innate in the child. Born in a remote Norfolk village, he may never have been the bright boy there, but he was never labelled educationally subnormal. He could manage. Let him move to London and the label may quickly attach itself to him. The number of classifications in school that are possible for children depends within these islands upon the size of the education authority and—not least—the efficiency of its transport. In the same Norfolk village, for example, the intelligent cerebral-palsied child may be ineducable and the dullard may paddle on with the rest.

Ineducable

The decision to 'ascertain a child as ineducable' may be taken at any time. The judgment which is made is a purely practical one: taking into account this child's assessable ability and the available educational provision, can he be educated here? It is important to understand the practical nature of the judgment when one is

[1] *Ibid.* p. 22.

considering the problem of the education of the child with cerebral palsy: this fact was recognised in the Education Act of 1944, for the responsibility to ascertain, which had formerly been the medical officer's, was by that Act placed squarely upon the education authority. The parents have a right of appeal to the Ministry and in the event of the appeal's failing they can ask for the child to be re-assessed at any time. The request is always granted, for no child may be excluded from school who is educable and a request that is made without substance betrays a miserable situation in which the parents have not accepted the reality; in such a situation help and advice, in the interests of both child and parents, must not be denied.

Occupation centres are provided by the local health authority for the ineducable. A distinction is drawn between the educability and the trainability of a child. For the purpose of this distinction education is regarded as beginning with reading, training with continence. If the child is reasonably continent, a patient attempt is made to train him in accepted social ways, to train his senses, to fill out his personality by means of painting, the use of colour, music and drama, to help him to follow some simple trade and to encourage any signs of educability. The child's attendance at a centre gives the mother much-needed personal relief. As with all handicapped children, the mental defective often proves to be more amenable outside his family circle, and the children all enjoy attending. This service began afresh after the war. There is now an established training scheme for the staff of the centres and a general feeling among them and others interested that a great deal more could be achieved if only more were known about methods of training and teaching the children and about the ways in which the group exerts its magic upon its members.

Some authorities will allow defectives to attend the centres up to any age, if they are unemployable. A large authority with efficient transport can classify its defectives in the centres by age and sex and within the centres by age and ability. Best progress is made in these circumstances. All authorities began by hiring make-shift accommodation, generally church halls. The more enter-prising have now built permanent centres and are experimenting with sheltered workshops. Some authorities are woefully slow to implement their statutory powers. Special mental health visitors are appointed to advise the parents and to assist with the many problems that arise for both the family and the defective child.

Special difficulties arise with both the physically and mentally handicapped who are in the higher grades when they reach school-leaving age: problems of working, earning money and forming relationships with persons outside the family and school groups arise, exacerbated by increasing physical needs, the desire for adult pleasures and possessions and the inability to compete at work.

The high-grade mental defective, especially, needs the opportunity to mature, emotionally and intellectually, at his own slow pace, and to receive training and guidance probably until his twenties. This is, unhappily, only forthcoming if he is in an occupation centre, when he is unlikely to be high-grade, and then only if he is in certain fortunate areas, or when he is certified, detained for an offence or—not later than eighteen years—when he is in care.[1]

J. F. MacMahon writes:

It is indisputable that the feeble-minded, under present-day conditions, owe their social inadequacy more frequently to defects of character and temperament than to intellectual inferiority.

Clinical observation suggests that the tardy blossoming of adolescent feeble-minded subjects as seen at this hospital is associated with their removal from unfavourable environmental conditions and the provision of training for them in new surroundings. Of course they cannot describe their childhood reactions to psychological traumata, but it seems probable that, in some instances, repressive or schizoid mechanisms contributed to their relatively poor test performances as well as to their social incompetence.

...among the sub-cultural nurture is so often decisive in determining the existence of high-grade defect, social competence, and the need for official action. Hence for purposes of diagnosis and prognosis it is futile to consider the moron apart from his environment, past, present, and future. In brief the chief function of mental deficiency practice (apart from the humane custodial care of low-grade cases) is to rescue impressionable young morons from adverse environmental conditions and to control their behaviour while they are being trained

[1] For an account of hopeful methods with feeble-minded adolescents see H. C. Günzburg, *Brit. J. Med. Psychol.* **30** (1957), 42.

to realize their mental and social potentialities. Thus when their characters have stabilised and they have achieved tolerable social competence at the close of their protracted psychological adolescence, it may prove possible to return them, not to environmental situations which proved disastrous for them, but to social conditions in the community likely to afford them fair prospects of fending for themselves and remaining useful citizens.[1]

Residential facilities

The doctor may recommend that the seriously handicapped be taught in special schools, either day or boarding. Whether the children are sent to schools of their own or those of voluntary societies, the education authority pays the fees. Some hospitals where children are in long-term care have hospital schools. There are two grammar schools for blind children, one for deaf children and growing provision for spastic children.

There is, it may be noted, a growing concensus of opinion that physically handicapped children—except possibly the blind—who are of normal or superior intelligence are poorly provided for. They may need special education because of their handicap but that ought not to mean education at a low intellectual level.[2] It is very difficult to find a placement for a child with a 'double handicap'. A child in a hospital without a hospital school, or at home, may be provided with a visiting teacher. In 1955 there were 120 hospital schools in England and Wales with 6476 children on the roll: 1425 other children were receiving individual tuition. The Ministry of Education in September 1956 asked local education authorities to review their arrangements for providing primary and secondary education for children in hospital and to see that they were as comprehensive as possible. The Minister of Health has asked hospitals to inform education authorities about the admission of any child likely to remain in hospital who is well enough for lessons.

The selection of the residential school or of the hospital to which a child is to go is not, of course, undertaken by the family doctor if the child is within the care of the local education authority. He

[1] *B.M.J.* **2** (1952), 254.
[2] See, for example, F. E. Schonell, *Educating Spastic Children* (Edinburgh, 1956).

may, however, advise on a private special school. Blind children must be sent to a residential school unless a special (and rare) exception is made by the Ministry. So, too, with rather more exceptions, must deaf children. The grounds on which residential schooling for the handicapped may be recommended must be considered. The first—and this is the reason why it is insisted that the blind and deaf receive resident schooling—is that some incurable defects can by intensive training and by association with other children with the same defect be effectively overcome. By means of prolonged treatment—orthopaedic, for example—other defects can be cured or remedied. Sometimes the defect or combination of defects is so gross that survival is possible only by institutionalisation. Or the rarity of the disease may make local day school provision impracticable. In yet other cases, in consideration of the handicap, the child's home may be unsatisfactory.

The handicapped child, his family and neighbourhood, must all be taken into account by the doctor when he is called on to advise. The burden at home may be damaging or intolerable. The removal of the child may be damaging to him, particularly if it is for custodial care. If he is to go to residential schooling with a real hope of return to normal life, he must face the break with his family, the adjustment to school, and, upon his discharge, the break with the school, his new role at home and readjustment to normal life. Hospitalisation will emphasise for some children their difference from others and upon their return, may have strengthened their determination to be different; for others it may be eagerly seized on as a way to gain confidence and ability to accept the challenge of everyday life. A child at a residential school may be able to acquire a means of earning a livelihood which might otherwise be denied him; another, unable to acquire the necessary skill, may return home a difficult, unemployable adolescent. For the individual case the individual judgment must be made. It may be added that whatever is done should be planned, so far as it is possible, with the knowledge and understanding of the child himself, for the greatest step is often the first: to obtain the co-operation of the child to cure or train himself.

Criticism

As long ago as 1932 A. Newsholme deprecated the separation of the infant-welfare and school-health services.[1] Professor A. Moncrieff has criticised school-health provision.[2]

1. They have changed little in thirty or forty years, and are still based on three routine inspections for the detection of defects and arrangement for their treatment.

2. Screening could be done by nurses and teachers as has been done in New York and Canada.[3] This observation has drawn adverse criticism from some correspondents, but similar criticism, if not necessarily a support for the same remedy, was forthcoming two years after Professor Moncrieff's from E. H. Wilkins: 'In every respect—accommodation, time allowed to each case, provision of medical equipment, method of recording, and lack of facility for research—the essentially medical character of the work has been submerged.'[4] Experiments upon the lines indicated have been conducted in Smethwick and West Bromwich. J. A. Lee[5] has reported that only 'about sixty per cent of the medical defects that cause the rejection of young men for military service are recorded on the documents of the School Health Service. This proportion is largely independent of the interval between the examinations at school and the pre-service examinations, and the discrepancies between the records are not limited to defects that might have developed in the interval. There is little information available about the effectiveness of the "periodic medical inspections" of the School Health Service, and there is need for their reassessment'.

3. The provision made for the handicapped child, is often very good but the provision for the ineducable does not reach the same standard.

4. The school medical officer should extend his activities to physical education, to the teaching of biology and of sex education, and to the study of the school as a healthy environment.

5. Care committees should be established in all areas.

The care committees are non-statutory bodies of voluntary workers, established only in London and entrusted by the London County Council's Education Committee, by whom they are constituted, with the duty of interesting themselves in the general

[1] *Medicine and the State* (London, 1932), pp. 41, 192.   [2] *B.M.J.* 2 (1950), 795.
[3] D. B. Nyswander, *Solving School Health Problems* (Commonwealth Fund and Humphrey Milford, 1942).
[4] *Medical Inspection of School Children* (London, 1952), p. 41.
[5] *B.M.J.* 1 (1958), 571.

welfare of the children in the Council's schools. Their aim is to promote the welfare of London school children through the education of their parents in the fullest possible use of the school services provided by both public services and voluntary organisations, so that each child may have every help in developing to his or her utmost capacity. Their responsibilities include:

1. Seeing that no child in need of food or clothing is unprovided for, either at home or through the school.

2. Ensuring that no child found by the school inspecting doctor, or dentist, to require treatment or advice, fails to receive it.

3. Ensuring that no child leaving school does so in ignorance of the possibilities the district has to offer in the way of further education and social recreation.

4. Investigating cases of children who appear neglected, and of children with behaviour problems, in need of child guidance, or other special treatments, in co-operation with other statutory or voluntary bodies.

5. Supplying information to the youth employment bureau before the school interviews, and co-operating with the youth employment officer in keeping in touch with young persons who for health, character or environmental reasons may need advice and help after leaving school.

6. Supplying information on cases referred to the petty sessions and on special housing problems.

They undertake house visiting and help in dealing with social problems of various kinds, such as illness and convalescence, lack of food and clothing, the lack of surgical and other requisites, and need for rest and holidays among the children and their families: this is done in conjunction with the appropriate statutory and voluntary agencies.[1]

They have been relieved of their former responsibilities with regard to employment, for the L.C.C. has exercised its powers and set up youth employment committees, as a separate service, incorporating these duties together with those formerly exercised by the Ministry of Labour with regard to the employment of juveniles (children under eighteen).

[1] The London County Council still maintain nutrition clinics to which are referred, it appears (L. H. Bell et al., Med. Off. 95 (1956), 163), children from 'problem families, or from families nearer the average where there are certain adverse factors, children with a history of serious operational illness, and children with a good social background with food fads, poor appetites, and other symptoms suggestive of emotional disturbances'.

CHAPTER X

THE HANDICAPPED
CHILD

It is being found increasingly helpful, as ideas change, to group together all 'exceptional children'. The term is used to include those with handicaps both physical and mental, together with the emotionally disturbed and the delinquent. Children who are a great deal brighter or more richly endowed physically than most are included within this concept, and, as we have seen, the idea is already being canvassed in Britain as the basis of the solution of educational problems which arise at the age of eleven plus. Perhaps the advantages of the term are that it enables common factors between these children to become clear, helps to rid thinking about the subnormal child of unhelpful emotional overtones, avoids the often quite accidental division between the disturbed and the delinquent and encourages the realisation that the super-endowed child has his own difficulties. Those children who occupy much of the doctor's time and thought are exceptional, for parents look for guidance in rearing their exceptional children. In this chapter consideration is given to the handicapped, but it is recognised that they can be best regarded as but one sub-group of exceptional children. The mentally handicapped are considered in most detail; there follows brief mention of the blind and deaf. Exhaustive treatment of the social aspects of handicaps in children is not attempted; but these two handicaps are included, first, to illustrate the common basic problems in dealing with handicapped children and, second, to point out something of the difficult problems of management that are involved. These two points have become of increasing relevance to the family doctor, for there is a growing questioning of the practice of sending such young children away from home. If the blind and deaf are to continue to be sent to the residential nursery, the task of preparing the child, in large part, may fall to the general practitioner; if they are to remain at home, he must have a skilled understanding of the rearing problems and be able to offer practical advice.

CHANGED ATTITUDE TO HANDICAPPED CHILDREN

Important factors in the changed attitude towards mental illness and defect and also, to some extent, towards permanent physical handicap, have been the mounting cost of institutionalisation, the difficulty of staffing the institutions available, the heavy pressure on existing accommodation and the growing realisation of the un-suitability of the available buildings, as interest in treatment and training have increased, together with an understanding that patients do better at home than in an institution. The current view is expressed by B. H. Kirman, who writes: 'The decision to place a child in an institution on account of mental defect is almost never in the child's interest; but it may be in that of another child or in that of the parents themselves.'[1]

The ascertainment of handicapped children is a statutory duty, laid upon the local education authority. It is increasingly realised that the early recognition of defect is of great importance and ought, for the happiness of the child and his family, but rarely to be delayed until schooldays. The control of some diseases has reduced the incidence of some forms of handicap but the reduction in infant mortality and in deaths from intercurrent infections in early childhood has also led to the survival of handicapped children who hitherto would have died. For example, D. F. Ellison Nash estimates that over the last fifteen years 'it seems likely that an average of 450 to 500 severe cases [of spina bifida] are being salvaged each year, these representing the group of children who would have died before the antibiotic era'.[2]

An impetus to British thinking was given by the work of A. Querido, Professor of Social Medicine at the University of Amsterdam, who, having been appointed city psychiatrist during

[1] *J. Mental Sci.* **99** (1953), 531.   [2] *B.M.J.* **2** (1956), 1333.

the economic depression of the thirties, was compelled to find some way of reducing the cost of mental disorder. His initial survey of institutions showed that ten per cent of the patients could be found a home, and the criterion became established that the decision whether or not a patient should be sent to an institution depended upon whether the consequences of the disease made it impossible for him to live in society.[1]

From there, he advanced to the stage of preventing new admissions. This was achieved by means of a centralised service, all admissions being made through the city psychiatrist who worked with a team available day and night to investigate on the spot: their main objective was to make the life of the patient tolerable and worthwhile in society. This domiciliary supervision was linked with facilities for clinical investigation in the university. The supervision was voluntarily submitted to and took place without warning. The uncooperative patient might, however, be sent to an institution.

Such a system is supported by sheltered workshops, foster-homes, funds for clothes and tools and means for finding employment. There is also direct relationship, by means of the sector-psychiatrist, with schools for the feeble-minded. Behaviour problems in children from normal schools are referred to the infant welfare clinics and the children's courts, and contact is maintained with their progress.

Changes in attitudes brought about by such work can be recognised throughout the *Report of the Royal Commission on Mental Illness and Mental Deficiency*.[2] It recognises three categories of mental disorder: mental illness, severe sub-normality (or mental deficiency) and psychopathy, and recommends the disuse of the terms 'of unsound mind' and 'feeble-minded'. Its prime concern in mental disorder is the sufferer's health and not the protection of society. It also recommends 'a general re-orientation away from institutional care in its present form and towards community care'. It looks to an expansion of local authority services, under medical officers of health, such as occupation and training centres, sheltered workshops, social centres and hostels. It seeks the

[1] *B.M.J.* 2 (1954), 1043.   [2] H.M.S.O. 1957.

abolition of the use of 'certification' and 'mental deficiency' and points out that as the law stands mental deficiency hospitals could drop all formalities for admission if they wished. The Minister has now acted on this (Circular 2158). Henceforward voluntary admission is the normal practice. Certification, leading to compulsory detention, is used only when this is considered essential for the protection of the patient or of the public.

It recommends that the provision of training for children who cannot benefit from the education provided in ordinary or special schools should continue to be the administrative responsibility of the local health authority rather than of the local education authorities, but that the present procedure of ascertaining children as 'ineducable' should be abolished and replaced by a procedure by which they would be 'recommended for training' in a training centre or hospital, just as children who need education in a special school are no longer 'certified', but 'recommended' for special forms of education.

The Commission was aware of the difficulty of organising training centres in rural areas, where it would be necessary to bring children from long distances, and it considered that residential training centres or residential homes for boarders near centres which were also attended by day pupils would be more helpful. Some children might be weekly boarders, others might stay for the equivalent of a school term.

PARENTS AND HANDICAPPED CHILDREN

There can be few more distressing duties for the doctor than to have to inform the parents that their child is permanently handicapped, whether it be physically or mentally or both. It is usual, says A. White-Franklin,[1] for parents to fail to notice that their baby is not normal 'even when parents include a doctor or a nurse'. The realisation that a child has an irremediable handicap places before the family doctor the fact that both he and the parents are presented with a permanent problem.

[1] *Lancet*, **I** (1958), 256.

The administrator, who deals in legally defined categories which provide him with labels for children, requires certainty before he will act: he is bound in the nature of things to err on the side of delay. The therapist is concerned less with categorical accuracy, and he realises that one named category shades off by imperceptible degrees into another and that, generally, the earlier treatment is commenced, the better. If doubts arise about a child in a doctor's mind, the sooner he squarely faces his own doubts the better for his personal comfort and for the success of the exercise of creating the best possible social and physical life for the child and his family. The doubt may be but momentary—say at the birth of a monstrous infant; it may, however, not arise for weeks, months or sometimes years. The less obvious the defect, the later the doubt arises, the more important it becomes to face it and not let it recede again.

When to tell the parents depends largely upon the physician's judgment of them: the object is for the parents to incorporate into their lives, into their thoughts and feelings, into their actions, into their whole way of life, as satisfactorily as possible, the fact that there is a permanent feature about the child which had not before been taken into account. It takes time for a couple to think and feel into the fact that a baby is on the way. It takes time to settle down with the baby, with the fact that it is a boy (or girl), with the fact that one is a father or a mother; and each one of us, more or less accurately, has at each stage our own way of feeling into a working relationship with the facts.

If the defect is obvious at birth, unless the condition of the infant makes it unavoidable, it is best not to attempt to tell the mother before one month is up. The early preparation of the father for the news is, however, to be advised.[1] The early mortality of low-grade aments may of itself resolve the problem. The doctor does not escape the responsibility, however, of having to prepare the parents for that possibility. The death of an infant of itself requires explanation to the western mind.

The mother must accept the facts: she must be helped to discover them herself. This does not mean either than she must be left in a

[1] R. S. Illingworth, in *B.M.J.* 2 (1955), 4.

fool's paradise or allowed to drag on anxiously and wearily with nagging doubts. Not only will she be angry with the doctor for not telling her before, but during the period of anxiety she will have been, at great expense to herself, a less efficient mother and wife. Some mothers, of course, are over-anxious: they expect their child to be a genius or at least to reach its milestones with a military precision. Such mothers are clearly in need of reassurance; but the problem in all cases is essentially the same: this woman is the mother of this baby—how best can they grow together? Advice—how simple and trite it sounds—is best received when people are ready for it. 'This is unpleasant, let's get it over quickly and cleanly and no nonsense about it', sounds humane and no doubt it is, if it *finishes* something: drains the boil, takes the nasty medicine. Do it quickly and it's over—we can forget it and go on with everyday life; the crisis is resolved. But the diagnosis of a handicap in a child finishes nothing: it begins an entirely new way of life for the parents. Most of us prefer a little preparation before we embark on something new. The family doctor may not be prepared to make the judgment alone, especially in border-line cases.[1] It is clearly wrong, however, that the mother should go blindly on until confronted by the paediatrician or the medical officer of health, for if the child is sufficiently unusual to merit being referred to them, he is so unusual that his parents ought to be prepared for the outcome of his examination. The final criterion of mental defect, as for any handicap, is a social rather than a clinical one.[2]

Some words and phrases should be avoided—'mental defect', 'mental', 'imbecile', 'feeble-minded', 'moron', 'idiot', 'there is nothing that can be done', 'for your sake I hope he dies', 'I cannot put a new head on your child's shoulders'. These words ought not

---

[1] Except for obvious idiots or imbeciles, the Ministry of Education Circular no. 146 (30 June 1947) recommends that children who are believed to be in-educable and are between the ages of two and five years should not be reported under Section 57 (3) of the Education Act 1944 until they have had a trial in an ordinary or special school.

[2] For illustration of this see the findings of N. O'Connor and J. Tizard (below, p. 205).

to be used to parents and certainly not 'hurled at them as if from an ambush'.[1] Preferable are 'backward', 'retarded', 'he will go at his own pace', 'he will need special care', 'I am interested in children with this handicap and we will rear and train him together'.

The problem is to get the parents to accept an inescapable fact. It is necessary, therefore, that they should be given time and encouragement to talk and ask questions. It is only thus that the doctor can have any inkling of his progress with the exercise which is the whole purpose of the interview. From their questions he can confirm or modify his judgment of their concepts and of their ability to understand.

If there is a bad family history, the parents may already be well-informed and their suspicions may have been aroused earlier than had been anticipated. If there is a positive explanation of the child's condition, the object must be to convey it to the parents. If it is possible to say that the condition is not due to infection, to inheritance, to birth injury or to bad obstetrical care, then say so. Distinguish, if appropriate, between insanity and defect. The parents need to know some idea of the prognosis: not only what the child will not be able to do, but also what he will be able to do. It is an enormous encouragement to parents to know that their baby will walk and talk, will be clean, will recognise them and love them as his Mum and Dad.

Sessions between the doctor and the parents may be time-consuming but they are rewarding. The family doctor is the best person to conduct them. Some hospitals, however, make special provision.

Generally paediatric staff consider it desirable for parents of children with chronic illnesses such as nephrosis or diabetes to have as much understanding as possible of the natural history of the disease, the rationale of diagnostic and therapeutic procedures, the relative significance of various symptoms, signs and laboratory examination and the essential problems in management.[2] As one

[1] K. Kanner, *Amer. J. Mental Deficiency*, **57** (1953), 379.
[2] See B. Korsch, L. Fraad and H. L. Barnett, *J. Pediatrics*, **44** (1954), 703.

of the methods of achieving this goal, paediatric discussions with parent groups have been held for the past several years in the New York Hospital Council Medical Center. The types of discussions varied and included series of three to five evening meetings each with parents of children with nephrosis and with diabetes mellitus. Since the psychiatric training of the paediatricians who led these discussions was limited, their function was nŏt that of psychotherapy. On the contrary, in the groups, as in their individual relationships with parents, the paediatricians served both as medical authorities and as physicians with whom the parents could work through some of their feelings about their sick children, their handling of them, and their relationship to the medical staff.

Parents' values

Success in situations of handicap largely turns upon the values of the parents. If in the mind of parents or physician the purpose of procreation is the production of the state scholar, the major-general or the millionaire, the outlook is obviously poor. It is worth pausing a moment, therefore, to remind ourselves what life may hold apart from social achievement. Listen to the headmaster of the great public school. Two things constantly recur in his pronouncements upon education and the success of his school in particular: First, that without a good home a boy is unlikely to succeed, and secondly, that, outstanding though the academic achievement of some boys may be, its importance is subordinated to the fact that every boy in the school grows within an atmosphere where the great values of life, of truth, beauty and goodness surround him and are instilled in him.

Now go to the occupation centre, where mentally defective children are brought together: children who will never pass the G.C.E.—who, in fact, will never read and write. What is there to give these children but the great values of life—truth, beauty and goodness?

Go on to the good family, to the mother with her infant and two toddlers—three boys being reared in the good home of which the headmaster approves and from which he will be glad to welcome the boys into his school. The mental ability of those boys at this stage may be on a par with, if not less than, that of the children at the occupation centre. Within this good home the children are lovable little boys, already nurtured in the ways of truth, beauty and goodness. The profound problems of education lie exposed in the nursery and in the occupation centre, stripped of the differential calculus and the Greek verbs. 'He is already a little person', says the mother of her infant. Except for the grossest, the handicapped, too, are already little persons.

Handicapped children can, whether their defect be mental or physical, grow into lovable persons, if there is love for them to experience and if that love can be conveyed to them in spite of their handicap. Psychotic idiot children progress wonderfully in an institution if they form an attachment to an understanding nurse only to relapse when the nurse leaves.[1]

The physical or mental handicap of a child may be so great that the mechanical problems of conveying to him the essentials of social life—be they food, love or speech—may be beyond the ability of parents and sometimes beyond the skill of the physician. Sometimes the revulsion of the parents and their misunderstanding of the child's needs may be so great that his potentialities remain unrealised. He may repel in others what he urgently needs and be unable to receive what comes his way. Communication is the fundamental problem in the lives of the handicapped. The neglected handicapped child is, when communication is meagre, sometimes to be compared to an animal.

From time to time there are stories of wolf-boys, antelope-boys, Mowglis, reared by animals. Few of the cases are well-documented, but they always rest upon the fact that the child's behaviour resembles the wolf's, resembles the antelope's, that he appears from an early age to have been subject to social pressures which are not human. No one denies that he has been without an environment: merely that he is a special case, and that therein lies the

[1] A. Repond, 'Reactions and Attitudes of Families towards their Physically and Mentally Handicapped Children' in *Family, Mental Health and the State* (W.H.O. 1955), pp. 2, 57.

interest. The latest such child to be recorded was picked up by the Lucknow police on 17 January 1954. A preliminary statement was made about him by Professor Kali Prasad.[1] He found a boy of nine or ten, starved, with a left hemiplegia, without callosities on his knees or his palms or his toes. It was obvious that he had never walked or stood up: he could neither walk on all fours nor even crawl. 'Ramu was probably abandoned as a helpless cripple by despairing parents who, having helped him to survive so long, eventually gave him up.' Physically defective, probably mentally defective too, this boy has lived for nine or ten years inter-active with and interdependent upon his environment. The boy's parents failed to teach him to walk, to feed, to talk. Not all mental defectives can be taught these things; but the suspicion is that it was because of the total inability of his family to nurture him that this boy, who showed an aversion to cooked foods, fruits and vegetables, accepted only raw meat.

Parents' reactions

(1) *Rejection*

Parents reactions may be to reject either the advice or the child; to attack the doctor, themselves, or the child; or to over-protect the child. Parents will have anxieties concerning other children, actual or potential, and will seek guidance about institutionalisation. Parents' reactions to the news are, of course, dependent upon their personality. They may reject the diagnosis—the doctor must be wrong, there is nothing wrong with the child—and be incapable of accepting the fact until an administrator is compelled to give his decision—for example, by ascertaining that the child is unable to benefit from schooling. It is sometimes inconceivable to European and North American parents that a disease or condition is incurable. This may lead them to abandon orthodox medicine altogether. 'God's will be done' is rarely heard in the surgery today. If the diagnosis is inescapable, they may reject the child—'I don't want to see it again. Take it away. It is horrible.' The unconscious

[1] K. Prasad, 'Ramu the Wolf Boy of Lucknow', in *Illus. London News* (27 February 1954).

hostility of one parent for another sometimes expresses itself in the rejection of a child who may in fact or fantasy resemble that parent.

Guilt feelings will be aroused and parents will seek to attribute blame. Was the doctor negligent in his supervision during pregnancy or at the confinement? Is it the husband's fault? Vaguely-heard talk is recalled and they begin to wonder—and the physician should be on the look-out for this—whether this is the penalty for alcoholism, syphilis, attempted abortion, a sexual aberration or perversion. 'I dropped the baby, doctor.' 'I fell when I was pregnant.' 'I went on working right to the end.' Personal fears and guilt are inevitably touched off. Weaknesses in personal relationships are strained: 'There's madness in your family.' 'Can it be my child?' 'I wonder what my wife was up to while I was away.' Parents and parents-in-law of the couple may be involved. 'His mother thinks I'm hopeless anyhow. She thinks I'm not good enough for him. She says it's because I don't manage the child properly. What will the neighbours say?' In the context of epilepsy W. G. Lennox writes what is also true of mental defect and is present to some extent in all handicaps:

An epileptic child brings psychologic and social complications for those around him which are subtle, severe and long lasting. Below and beyond the family is the widening substructure of friends, school-teachers, acquaintances, and the general public. The conception of epilepsy which resides in the public mind is most important. For centuries the pyramid of therapy has had a foundation not of masonry but of rubble and sand.[1]

Anxiety and guilt may lead the parents to blame anyone associated with the child: 'He was perfectly all right till he went to hospital for appendicitis. I don't know what happened but he has never been the same since.' 'He was frightened by his brother letting off a firework. They let them run about wild at school. He knew his letters when he went to school; now he doesn't know a thing. It's the school. They keep him cooped up there. All the children are frightened of Miss Blank. Of course he doesn't learn.'

Anxiety and guilt may lead the parents to blame and attack the

[1] *J. Pediatrics*, **44** (1954), 591.

child. The diagnosis is rejected and blame may be put upon his body—his tonsils, hearing, vision—or upon himself. An organised attack may then be instituted upon the organs of his body, or a system of discipline or training instituted, rising, in despair—especially with the lethargic or weak child—from constant nagging to coercion, beating and finally brutal assault. 'It's nothing more than that, he is lazy, doesn't pay attention, isn't interested.'

D. A. Pond and B. Bidwell say that a number of mothers of *petit-mal* children show an astonishing contempt of their weakly passive youngsters. The mothers have high and rigid standards and 'there is a subtle rejection of these children by their parents and these family stresses may be so severe that the child has to be removed to an epileptic colony before treatment is successful.'[1]

(2) Over-protection

The passionate attachment of a mother to a handicapped child that gives her the certainty that she alone understands him must not be mistaken for the desired relationship. Her passion is fed by an ambivalent flame in which anxiety or guilt, or both, are major factors, and the child will warp in its heat. Of the apparently desirable sentiments, the expressed feeling that the handicapped child is particularly the parents' own, that he will always be their baby, that he will never grow, needs some consideration by the family doctor. A babied child will remain a baby, and in the long run, when the parents are old, infirm or dead, that may not be a desirable role. Some adult defectives and other handicapped persons are nursed throughout their lives exclusively by their mothers. The death of the parent or temporary separation from her becomes an often unnecessarily heavy blow. It is as well, for this reason if no other, to persuade the mother to share her burden.

(3) Other children

The parents will want to know about having another baby, about the chances that it will be normal. The doctor may well find that the couple are disinclined to have intercourse, unable to face

[1] *B.M.J.* **2** (1954), 1522.

the possibility of there being another child. Genetic questions inevitably arise. There are now, following the work of Professor Tage Kemp in Copenhagen, genetics-counselling clinics in London, Leeds, Bristol and Liverpool.

Parents will ask about the effect upon normal children in the family. Does it matter having him with the other children? The question can only be answered for the individual family.

Fred, aged six, is the youngest son of a successful young army officer. His elder brother, aged eight, is a mongol. The mother is devoted to the mongol, who is a nice, well-behaved little boy who occupies nearly all her attention. Fred is a timid, rather negative, tearful lad.

Father was delighted with Fred at his birth. Both parents were immensely relieved that he was normal and another boy. Father urges Fred to do things beyond his powers and is angered by his tears and timidity.

(4) Institutionalisation

Parents are bound to seek guidance about sending the child to an institution. The inquiry may be based primarily upon the rejection of the child or upon the practical impossibility of managing him.

The nursing problem presented by all except the most severely handicapped infants is much the same as for the normal infant and toddler. It is seldom or never in the interests of the child to be put into an institution. All handicapped children do best when their daily experience is as near as possible to normal life. The degree of defect will clearly influence the decision, but unless that is gross then from the infant's point of view there is no hurry: he is not to be rushed off to begin a therapeutic process as soon as possible.

Private home accommodation is expensive, and parents may sometimes, for that reason, be the more prone to seek it. Public provision, except for the emergency, is not easy to come by. Parents may place their children in an institution and 'forget about them'. Every superintendent is responsible for dozens of patients who never receive a visit, a present or a post-card. Parents are encouraged to visit their children, may take them out and may have them home for visits. Mental hospital authorities, attempting to meet a demand for places beyond their ability and believing a child does better at home than in the hospital, will not discourage parents from having their children home. Parents are sometimes horrified to find that their child has made a good adaptation to the hospital and when taken out or taken home makes it quite plain that he prefers the hospital.

The decision to institutionalise is, however, one that the parents must take themselves. It is also one that cannot be avoided, for parents early realise that provision must be made against their own incapacity by age and their eventual death. The recurring questions are: 'Is it fair to burden the other children as we have been burdened?' 'Haven't his brothers and sisters had to bear sufficient burden?' 'Would their chances of marriage be imperilled?' 'Would their spouses refuse to have the defective "child"?'

In a survey by N. O'Connor and J. Tizard, the authors found that about half the mental defectives under statutory care were above imbecile level.[1] Social factors are more important than lack of cognitive ability when it comes to living and working among normal people. G. McCoull and L. Slupinski, however, found in one hospital in Northumberland classification at variance with that of O'Connor and Tizard.[2]

	No. of cases under investigation	Idiots		Imbeciles		Feeble-minded	
		No.	%	No.	%	No.	%
O'Connor and Tizard	592	35	5·9	247	41·7	310	52·3
Present series	1011	246	24·3	509	50·3	256	25·3

If the 'sample figures' produced by O'Connor and Tizard give a true account of the actual population of the twelve mental deficiency hospitals under review [say McCoull and Slupinski] then it would appear that there are marked differences in approach to the question of mental defectives in hospital and perhaps different criteria concerning the function which a mental deficiency hospital is supposed to serve.

[1] N. O'Connor and J. Tizard, *B.M.J.* 1 (1954), 16; and (more fully) N. O'Connor and J. Tizard, *The Social Problem of Mental Deficiency* (London and New York, 1956).
[2] G. McCoull and L. Slupinski, *B.M.J.* 2 (1954), 341.

Today the trend of opinion is summarised by L. Hilliard:

Mental deficiency practice has consolidated within the framework and experience of an Act designed forty years ago in very different social circumstances. This has resulted in a wastage of human capabilities which I believe can, in more favourable circumstances, be developed and utilised to better advantage both to the individual and to the community. Mental deficiency of the so-called feeble-minded category is in many cases not a clear-cut clinical entity of an irreversible nature. Too often, as I have tried to show, it is the diagnosis which has created the disease.[1]

Management of handicapped children

The object of management is to permit the child to lead his own small life and to take his own place within the family. Handicapped children can generally achieve more than their parents will permit, for in their over-anxiety and guilt they often spoil their children. By going at the child's pace, which the parent has to learn, his independence is to be achieved. Even when the explanation to the parents is successful and they are able and willing to accept that their child is permanently handicapped, even so they are bound to ask the question, 'What can we do?'

When the parents fully understand the situation, they will be eager to put all their energy into providing for their handicapped child. It is no good simply telling the mother to love him, or to take him to the infant welfare centre. This is a very special child— the doctor has told her so—and she looks for special provisions. Where, as for example in epilepsy or diabetes, there is treatment, the parents may be worried about the very treatment and need reassuring about the risk of their child's becoming a 'drug-addict'. With the diabetic 'a disciplined way of life is an essential therapeutic requirement. This is easily achieved in the intelligent child bred in a good home, but even there it demands co-operative parents and continued care by an interested and instructed doctor.'[2] The ordinary social welfare facilities are available, of course, for the parent. The National Assistance Board may make alterations in the home—ramps, wider doors, appliances and special furniture—

[1] *B.M.J.* 1 (1954), 1374.   [2] *B.M.J.* 2 (1954), 1536.

so that the handicapped child may live more comfortably and more efficiently.

At any time after the child is two, the parents may ask to have him examined to see if he requires special educational treatment. The local education authority is bound to examine and any necessary special facilities must be provided if the parent wishes.

The mental health visitor of the local health authority should early establish herself as a friend of the family where there is a mentally handicapped child. She will introduce the mother to the occupation centre, or if that is not possible or desirable, to the home teacher, to the facilities for 'short-stay' in the event of illness at home or of the mother's needing a prophylactic holiday, and, where possible, for holidays for the handicapped child. Some relief from the child during the day is of benefit to the mother; longer relief—a summer holiday—may be of great importance. Without her, her child, whether at home or in a 'short-stay' home, is not likely to do so well as in her company. The mother must be prepared so that she realises that the child's discomfort is an inevitable part of the price that has to be paid for her necessary respite.

Parents' associations

The parents ought to be introduced to the parents' association for the particular handicap. From membership of the association, parents derive considerable comfort and support, and the associations perform a real social service in contributing to the health of the whole family group. Similar support comes from membership of 'friends of hospitals'. ·

It is useful to have the literature of the associations available to give to parents at the earliest appropriate opportunity. It is often the first indication they have that there are other parents with similar problems and, sometimes, merely to see a reference in a pamphlet to children like their own is an extraordinary comfort.[1]

---

[1] *Rehabilitation Literature, 1950–55* (National Society for Crippled Children and Adults, London, 1957) lists 5214 articles, pamphlets and books on medical care, education, employment, welfare and psychology of handicapped children and adults.

The service of the associations to their members is perhaps best understood if some of the foregoing considerations are now recounted from the point of view of the parents of a mentally defective child. The mother takes her infant to the doctor, unhappy about its progress. The doctor has at some time to tell her that the child is defective and incurable. Gently but clearly—clearly it must be, for he does not want to raise false hopes—he tells the mother that nothing can be done for her child. Her immediate—almost logical—reaction is to say that the doctor must be wrong. Doctors cure illness, doctors study disease. There must be an answer and someone must know. She goes, then, from doctor to doctor; from doctor to hospital; from hospital to hospital; from hospital to quack and from quack to quack.

Impoverishment of social and family life

The doctor must tell her that mental defect happens for the most part we know not how or why, that it happens to the Pole as to the Portuguese, to the American as to the British. 'It is not your fault.' The mother's immediate response will probably be, 'Then, if it is not my fault, is it the fault of my husband?' The doubt, once it is aroused, is not easily allayed and it does not provide comfortable thoughts for the couple to share by their fireside in the evening.

The mother takes her child out for his daily airing. People glance at the ugly child, ill-controlled, perhaps noisy; they glance, they feel surprise if not horror, and look away quickly. The result is the mother ceases to take her child out. At home her child is ugly, ill-controlled, perhaps noisy. Visitors are uncomfortable and so they cease to have people home. The social life of the family becomes confined to the dwelling; its participants are the parents and perhaps a normal child or two. Their life is restricted, thin and poor. Lonely and anxious, angry, they know not why, there is always at the back of the parents' minds the question, 'What happens to this child of mine when I die?' Emotions become entangled. The defective may suffer the shattering affection of his parents and also be the object of their hate—recognised or unrecognised. The normal children lead restricted lives and find their own emotions confused. For the parents merely to meet other parents with a similar child is a revelation and comfort, because the first defective child most people recognise is their own. To get them to meet older parents who are shouldering their difficulties and, indeed, an old couple who have made a satisfactory adjustment, is markedly therapeutic.

When the different sets of parents come together, they can be encouraged to organise practical help for each other—baby-sitting, outings, and so on. 'I haven't been on holiday or out for the day', mothers will say, 'for years. People stare, he is always sick in a car and then he is worse-behaved. It's more trouble than it's worth.' Together, however, the parents can hire a coach, and if her child is sick, it doesn't matter much because her neighbour's is too, and altogether the adults are used to defective children. On the beach they will make a group large enough to be self-centred, so that the parents can be at ease without taking into account the normal families.

It is not long, however, before they begin to quarrel. Poor in social relationships and anxious as they are, their quarrelling is cathartic and to be expected, but it is not always easy to manage. A later stage is for parents to organise themselves 'against'. It must be 'against' something, for the organisation is essentially aggressive: against the local health authority, the Regional Hospital Board, the Board of Control, the Ministry of Health. The object is to obtain better conditions for their children. No one can doubt that there is a great deal that can be done to improve all aspects of provision for the handicapped: but the really effective result is in quite other terms—it is the personalisation of the anonymous bureaucratic machines within which the parents are inevitably enmeshed. In response to an irritable and possibly demanding letter, a physician-superintendent, an administrator from the Board of Control will sit down and discuss the difficulties with the parents. The parents will discover that within the machine are ordinary men and women and that many, if not all of them, are keen on their jobs. It will call for a high degree of insight and understanding on the part of the officials to play their part. In effect they are called upon to make a psychiatric judgment as to how far the matter under discussion is determined by objective fact and how far by the subjective burden of the parents—and to give equal, if different, consideration to both aspects.

Emotional improvement

A mature stage is reached when parents seek to combine so as to co-operate with those professionally concerned with mental defect, when they begin to understand the possibilities of scientific investigation and find for themselves within it a co-operative role.

These things—outings, meetings, quarrels—may sound small to the point of insignificance. But we are considering the happiness, social efficiency, indeed the very physical health of people, members of a handicapped family. If these things are to be improved, then it cannot be by the drug, the knife, the apparatus: happiness, social efficiency and health can only be improved by the magic that is within the group.[1]

BLIND CHILDREN

That a child is blind is likely to be discovered at home and the family doctor will be involved in the child's early training. The problem is to rear him so that he is self-reliant. The parents have to come to understand that the child, never having seen, or having seen for but a short time, is not 'deprived': that he has his own life to live, though it is different from that of a sighted person, and that robust physical and mental development is possible without vision. Parents may manage better if they have already reared a baby and know from experience what the sighted child can do. They ought, anyhow, to be acquainted with the 'milestones' so that they may have some estimate as to what 'self-reliance' means at a given age. The parents ought early to be put in touch with the local blind association and to visit a Sunshine Home and a residential school so

---

[1] For a review of parent-guidance see J. H. Levy, *Exceptional Child*, **19** (1952), 1, 19.

that they may know what can be achieved, and come to accept the residential school as desirable. To do well there, the child must be emotionally well developed. He will leave home for resident care early by any standards and this development is, therefore, the more important to cultivate. The general practitioner should be alerted by weaning difficulties (not uncommon among blind children) for over-protection or rejection of the baby by the mother.

Particular attention within the house must be given to the common causes of accidents to children and the dangers must be removed. The child is much more dependent upon hearing and touch than the sighted child for the exploration of the outside world, and he ought, therefore, to be as much as possible in the company of an older sighted person, be provided from his earliest days with a wide range of things to handle and be encouraged to explore by touch.

Parents have a great deal to learn. For example they sometimes have difficulty in getting their infant, blind from birth, to sit up and stand. This may well indicate that they have accepted the line of least resistance and are bringing things to the child—over-protecting, pampering him—rather than encouraging him to go out and get things. If he has been too long in the cot, the child will throw back his head when his mother calls, for that is where mother's voice comes from—above. If he is held under his shoulders, dandled to walk, his head goes back again, for again mother's voice comes from above. If mother's voice were across the room, he would go towards it. Some blind babies move backwards at first rather than forwards when crawling, and they should not be discouraged from doing so. Parents sometimes complain that their blind—and particularly deaf and blind—children sleep little. Certainly such children cannot tell night from day by sight, but a sufficiently active and regular routine will provide its own rhythmic demand for sleep.

Blind babies, toddlers and children should be given as much airing as sighted children, and they should play with other children as much as possible. 'Reins' are very useful for training the blind child to walk, and especially for teaching curb drill.

Calm parents are perhaps the greatest asset a handicapped child can have. It is not easy for them to see his explorations to understand the 'clues' he learns, or watch his failure. But many handicapped children acquire the same ability to tumble which is slowly (and painfully) acquired by adults when they are taught Judo.

If the child is mentally normal, he ought to be able to walk at the usual age, go up and downstairs, use the lavatory, wash, dress and undress himself, eat and drink, though he may use a spoon for eating rather than a knife and fork longer than a sighted child, and buttons are not easy for him to manage.

Exploration by touching is an active progress; seeing is relatively passive. We see all the time our eyes are open. Hearing and smelling and skin perception are similar to seeing in that they too are passive and the child must be encouraged to take interest in all three. This requires the parents to hear, smell and feel the world anew. Blind babies and children generally enjoy their bath because of the noises and smells and the skin stimulation, and the parents may often learn new insights into the child's world by helping his explorations in a leisured bath.

With hearing comes speech; but speech is also learned by looking at people's faces and particularly mouths. The blind child cannot do this and his speech may well be faulty not because he is either deaf or stupid, but because he cannot see. Because his appearance does not matter to him, because he never learns the visual norms, it may be necessary to train him not to roll his eyes or grimace and to sit and walk in accepted ways. Some blind children protect their faces as they move about. As their confidence grows, it becomes possible to teach them to keep their arms down.

At some time a child comes to realise that other people have a means of dealing with the environment denied to him. At first he may regard this facility merely as another attribute of adulthood: but he may well come to fear it. Here in reality is the 'being watched' of paranoia, the all-seeing God of some religions. The parents have to be prepared to explain this difference and to name it. For the parents, then, there will be a similar series of difficulties as for the physician in explaining the handicap originally. Moreover, there is the factor of personal involvement. Telling the child is one of the greatest tests of the parents of the blind.

The mere fact that the child is blind does not inevitably provide him with emotional and behaviour difficulties. Accepted by his family as a complete person, taking his place within the family, neither at the centre nor on the periphery, he may be as contented as any other child. 'A harsh, uncertain, or over-protective parent with extreme ideas about "normality" may easily lead to the child's perception of himself as one who is inferior and unable to deal with his environment. He will then behave as if he were inadequate....'[1] The use of visual words does not necessarily imply faulty rearing or betray a compensatory mechanism: he hears speech and may take over, for example, 'blue sky' because the two words go together, just like a small boy who corrected his mother at the point-to-point: 'No not winners, Mum; let's pick the bloody winners, like Wag.'

It is a pity if the blind infant develops badly. There are fewer blind now than hitherto, the services available are more comprehensive than for any handicap, and the skill and goodwill available to assist are very large, from birth through childhood to education and employment. Just as examples, there are blind undergraduates, lecturers and professors.

Facilities

The county councils and county borough councils are compelled by the Minister under the National Assistance Act to make arrangements for the welfare of persons who are blind. This is in addition to the facilities that must be provided by the education authority, and mainly refers to adults. There are many hostels, homes, residential nurseries and special schools run by voluntary associations in addition to those provided by the local authorities. Information concerning these and advice generally can be obtained from the Royal National Institute for the Blind. The Institute has newly established a parent unit in South Devon where a mother, her blind child and, if necessary, other members of the family may stay so

[1] L. Myerson, 'A Psychology of Impaired Hearing' in W. M. Cruikshank (ed.), *Psychology of Exceptional Children and Youth* (London, 1956), p. 162.

that the mother may be trained to manage her child. Mothers are ordinarily allowed to take their children to the school or nursery and may spend a night or two there. Arrangements are generally made for children to be able to speak to their parents by telephone.

There are home teachers for the blind who are examined by the College of Teachers of the Blind and appointed either by local authorities or voluntary associations. They undertake, among other things, the training and care of the pre-school child and of the school child on holiday, general welfare work, and the training of the deaf and blind.

DEAF CHILDREN

Although 'the family doctor can do more than anyone else to secure early diagnosis and treatment',[1] the young deaf child presents the family doctor with certain difficulties, mainly that of distinguishing him from the mentally backward. Deaf babies may develop more or less normally until they are eighteen months old, when the babbling of the normal child turns to speech. The need of diagnosing deafness as soon as possible is recognised, so that ideally both mother and child may be trained together. A hostel for that purpose has been established at Ealing, and by 1954 there were pre-school clinics for deaf children in Manchester, Birmingham, Leicester, Newcastle on Tyne and London. All have training facilities. By early 1958 there were at least forty-two audiology clinics.[2] Deaf aids for young children are available through the health service. Their use requires skilled technical advice. They magnify not only speech but all sounds, distort some speech sounds and give no indication of the location of sound.

There are many degrees of defect from complete deaf-mutism to a defect so slight that it can be detected only by special tests. Children with severe defects may have 'islands of hearing', and they become aware of vibrations and the movement of air in a

[1] *Ministry of Health Memorandum on the Prevention and Alleviation of Deafness* (H.M.S.O. 1957).
[2] J. B. Perry Robinson, *Report for the National Deaf Children's Society on the Care of the Deaf* (London, 1958).

manner rarely, if ever, cultivated by the hearing; they become aware, too, of small visual signs. It must not be forgotten that, without hearing, knowledge of the environment is disjointed: people and things creep up silently from behind—and suddenly are there. When deafness is discovered, the family problems are similar to those arising from other handicaps. The parents have to learn to communicate with their child. There is, however, probably less agreement among the experts as to how this is to be accomplished than, for example, in dealing with the blind child. If he can see, the child understands that speech is a means of communication, and the problem is to link speech with vision. Parents must be encouraged to speak to and with the child, to create the 'child-talking atmosphere', encouraging the use of what hearing he has, his ability to vocalise, and the linking of these with the body and facial movements of others. If the child's vision is impaired there are particular difficulties, for the child's energies may be fully devoted to visual exploration. Generally, skilled help is then necessary.

With normal children, the 'look and say' method is now commonly used to teach reading. Normal children are taught to recognise whole words and to say them long before they can spell them. Children are taught to recognise words in places other than in their reading books by seeing labels with the word written large on many objects in the classroom. They are taught to look at the word, just at one might at a hieroglyph or a drawing and to say what it represents—table, blackboard, waste-paper basket. In this method hearing plays a relatively minor role, and it can therefore be developed with success for use with deaf children. Some mothers can successfully teach their three-year-old deaf children a few essential words. The deaf are obviously more dependent upon the written word than the hearing and the child's interest in reading should be encouraged. In turn, the child's interest in words, in vocalisation, and in lip movements reinforce each other. Close co-operation between parent and teacher is necessary in order to see that they use a common vocabulary and that both keep pace with the extension of the child's knowledge of words.

All this must be achieved without fuss, without undue demands being made on the child, for, as L. Myerson has said, 'To live up to the demands of others when they are inappropriate may require that the person blunt his experiences, restrict his awareness of reality, and develop a self that is shadowy and superficial.'[1] Furthermore, the deaf child, like other handicapped children, may because. of a misunderstanding of his needs not only present his parents with the common 'negative phase' as a three-year-old, but may add to that a fiercely aggressive reaction to his frustrations and become unmanageable. That these difficulties are environmentally induced is demonstrated by a striking reversal reported by A. Repond. He tells of isolated backward Swiss families living in clans among whom there is congenital deaf-mutism. With them, he says, the birth of a deaf child—often illegitimate—presents no difficulties. It is upon those adults who can hear, especially if the child has his hearing, that rearing falls. The deaf-mute parents fail with the hearing child after its early infancy, and the children become very difficult; but the deaf children do not present difficulty and he knows of no paranoia of the deaf demanding hospitalisation among the clans.

Children cannot be considered apart from their environment. The handicapped child born in Cornwall produces different problems from that born in Cumberland or Camberwell; different problems arise among the Browns from those among the Smiths. The problems and their differences can be dismissed or ignored only at the risk of human waste and damage.

Facilities

There are, to summarise, a good many facilities which may be mobilised to support the home where there is a permanently handicapped child. Apart from those facilities which may be provided from two onwards by the education authority (see p. 207), equipment and structural alterations are forthcoming from the National Assistance Board (p. 206), the local health authority may provide home nursing and home helps (p. 115), together with

[1] *Op. cit.* p. 71.

advice, supportive visits and the loan of equipment (p. 162), the special visitors (pp. 158 and 207), the home teachers (p. 188) and the self-help societies (p. 207).

Among the facilities available are also the voluntary societies, of which the Invalid Children's Aid Association is among the most important. This society provides assistance and advice to sick and crippled children and their parents, supplementing the provisions of the National Health Service Act. It maintains recuperative holiday homes, residential schools of recovery, pays for special holidays and diets, and gives immediate help for many children whose requirements may later be met under the Act, to avoid unnecessary delay and suffering. It provides a bureau of information about existing facilities for the treatment of children and those needs for which no provision has yet been made; and offers practical training in social work for university students, health visitors and social workers. There are thirty branches in Greater London.

There are local societies of the deaf—now considering associating themselves together into a national federation. The National Institute of the Deaf, Gower Street, London, W.C. 1, provides information.

Mere referral to the agencies can at the worst be the avoidance of a permanent problem by the family doctor; at the best it can mean he is bringing into play a useful partner in the co-operative venture between parents and the interested and instructed doctor.

INDEX

Abandoned child, 138–40
Accidents, 26, 118–21, 157
Accidents in the Home, Report of the Interdepartmental Committee, 119
Acta Endocrinologica, 14 n.
Adler, A., 65
Adoption, 76, 126–9
  Adoption act (1950), 125
  guardian *ad litem*, 129
  National Insurance Act Allowance, 138
  order, 128
  Report of the Departmental Committee on the Adoption of Children, 124
  society, 126
Alexander, W. P., 177
American Journal of Mental Deficiency, 198
Amulree, Lord, 120, 121
Annual Abstract (1957) of Statistics, 112
Approved lodgings, 78
Approved school, 79, 82
Approved school order, child 'in care', 139
Assumptions and beliefs, 38–40
Attendance centre, 81

Baker, A. E. (ed.), *William Temple and his Message*, 178
Baker, D. M., 'Physical Education and the Health of the Child', 175
Banks, A. L., 147
Bell, L. H., 191
Beyond control, 76, 82
Birth certificates, 'shortened', 125
Blind, 184, 188, 189, 192, 210–14
Blishen, E., 178
Boarding out, 130, 138, 139, 140
Borstal, 80
Bowlby, J., *Maternal Care and Mental Health*, 43
Brain, Sir Russell, 111
British Journal of Educational Psychology, 31, 181

British Journal of Medical Psychology, 65 n., 187 n.
British Journal of Preventive and Social Medicine, 153
British Journal of Psychology, 174 n.
British Journal of Social Medicine, 118
British Journal of Sociology, 125
British Medical Association, 142
British Medical Journal, 7, 14, 18, 20, 27, 41, 44–5, 84, 94–6, 106, 111, 118, 119, 120 n., 120, 121, 131, 143, 152, 155, 156, 157, 160, 161, 164, 188, 190, 193, 194, 196, 203, 205, 206
Browne, F. J., 153 n.
Bryant, H., 151
Burns, John, 147, 156
Burt, Sir C., 31, *The Backward Child*, 53, 174 n.

Care and protection, 76, 82, 187
  'after-care', 140
  care committee, 183, 190–1
  local authority duty to receive lost and abandoned children, 138, 139; co-ordinating committee, 146
Care of Children, Report of the Committee on the, 139
Carruthers, G. B., 131
Cassel, J., 'A Comprehensive Health Program among South African Zulus', 27
Catholic Marriage Advisory Council, 98, 131
Child guidance clinic, 98, 102–6
Child minders, 137
Children Act (1948), 138
Children and Young Persons (Amendment) Act (1952), 142
Children's nursing unit, 160
Children's officer, 77, 139, 146
Clark, M. M., *Left-handedness*, 57
Colebrook, L., 121
Colebrook, L., Colebrook, V., Bull, J. P. & Jackson, D. M., 120

Craig, W. G., Kitching, G. A., Davies, I. G. & Fraser Brockington, C., 161
Creak, E. M., 20
Crew, F. A. E., 119
Cruelty, 82, 141
Cruelty to and Neglect of Children, 142, 147
Cruikshank, W. M. (ed.), *Psychology of Exceptional Children and Youth*, 213, 215–16
Culture conflict, 15, 52, 60, 63

Day nursery, 137, 163
Deaf child, 184, 189, 192, 214–17
pre-school clinic, 214
Demands, 25, 32–5
Detention centre, 80–1
Discharge, conditional and unconditional, 78
District nurse, 160
see also Home nursing
Divorce
and children, 132–4
National Insurance Act Allowance for Child, 138
and separation, 132–4
Douglas, J. W. B. & Blomfield, J. M., *Children Under Five*, 118, 119, 157
Dykes, R. M., *Illness in Infancy*, 156

Education
child not receiving efficient, 83, 88
duty of parent to provide, 165–6
extrinsic and intrinsic, 60, 61, 178–9
further, 170, 191
Ministry of, 168–9
permissive and authoritarian, 61–6
physical, 175
remedial, 103
Educational Reconstruction, 86
Educational treatment, duty to provide, 207
Educationally subnormal, 176, 184, 185
see also Subnormal child
Eleven-plus, 173–5, 192
Ellis, R. W. B., 'Puberty and Adolescence', 180
Ellison Nash, D. F., 193
Employment and handicapped child, 187, 189
Employment of children, 88, 167–8
youth committees, 191

Encounter, 10
Enquire Within, 34
Ethics, 29, 30
Exceptional Child, 210
Expectation of life, 112
Expectations, 25, 36

Family Allowance, 110, 138, 147, 160
Family
and handicapped child, 98–100, 186–7, 189, 195–217
culture and tradition, 29–45
extended, 113
immediate, 109–10, 112
incompetent, 144–9
ineffective, 141–4
limitation, 110–12
nuclei, 108
passive learning in, 29–45
primary needs, 29
problem, 141–9; and local authorities, 145–6; Ministry of Housing attitude, 146
social life impoverished, 208
Family, Mental Health and the State, 62, 200, 216
Family Planning Association, 111
Family Service Units, 147–8
Family Welfare Association, 132
Fathers
and the birth of a defective child, 196
and corporal punishment, 72–3
and divorce, 133
family relationships, 31–2, 54, 93, 102
Ferguson, S. M. & Fitzgerald, H., *Studies in the Social Services*, 116
Fines, 79
Fisher, Mrs. G., 147
Fit person order, 79, 82
Folkways, 29, 30, 33
Forces Help Society, 137
Ford, D., *The Deprived Child*, 91
Foster-mother, 125
Fostering, 129–30, 139, 158
Fox, W. G. & Collins, F. D. O., 36
Freud, S., 12, 64
Friends of hospitals, 207
Froebel, 54, 55, 61, 63

Gallagher, M., 180
Geddes, J. E., 155

General Practice
  and adoption, 126
  and blind child, 193, 210–14
  and case-work agencies, 217
  and child guidance service, 102, 106
  and child welfare clinics, 152
  and cruelty, 141
  and deaf, 193, 214–17
  and domiciliary care of premature
    infants, 162; of sick children, 160–2
  and explanation and advice, 18–20,
    84–106
  and family group homes, 140
  and folklore, 50
  and gifted children, 87–8, 192
  and 'good' children, 85
  and grouped cottage homes, 140
  and handicapped child, 99, 188–9,
    192–217
  and the health visitor, 152, 158–9
  and home hazards, 121
  interchange of information with
    hospital board, 183
  interchange of information with
    school health service, 183
  and the local maternity and child
    welfare authority, 152
  and local norms, 31–45
  and neighbourhood, 21–8
  and parents associations, 207–8
  and parents of handicapped children
    99, 195–217
  and problem families, 141–9
  and punishment, 67
  and the Queen's Nurse, 160
  and residential provision for handi-
    capped child, 188–9
  and schooling, 66, 88, 163, 182
  and sexual irregularities, 100–2; see
    also Incest; Sexual offences against
    children
  and the therapeutic relationship,
    88–94, 94–6, 96–102
  and the unmarried mother, 123
Genetics counselling clinics, 204
Gibbens, T. C. N. & Walker, A.,
  Cruel Parents, 143
Gifted child, 87–8, 192
Gillet, J. A., 160 n.
Glass, D. V. & Grebenick, E., Trend
  and Pattern of Fertility in Great
  Britain, 122

'Good' Children, 85–6
Greenland, C., 122
Guardian, unable to exercise, or not
  exercising, proper care, 82, 138
Guardians allowance, 138
Guardianship, 135
Günzburg, H. C., 187 n.

Handicapped child, 192–217
  changed attitude to, 193–5
  and employment, 187, 189
  expected frequencies, 184
  and family, 98–100, 186, 195–217
  management of, 206–7
  National Assistance Board, 206
  parents and, 195–217
  parents' reactions to, 201–4
  provision for, of superior intelli-
    gence, 188
  residential provision, 188
  school health service responsibility
    from two, 156
  social factors in classification, 184,
    194, 197, 205
  special provision for, 184–9
  see also Educationally subnormal;
    Ineducable; Mental defect; Nur-
    sery, residential; School, residen-
    tial education; Subnormal child
Hansard, 119, 121
Harvey, A., 'Operation Pavement',
  116 n.
Head Teachers' Review, 171
Health Visiting, Inquiry into, 158
Health visitor, 158–60
  and general practice, 158–9
  hospital attendance, 161
  mental, 207
  and problem families, 146, 148
Hewitt, D. & Stewart, A., 118
Hilliard, L., 206
Hobson, W., 7
Home
  childless, 126–30
  dependent, 116
  disturbed or broken, 130–41
  exceptional types of, 114–49
  help, 115, 158, 162, 216
  help and problem families, 148
  inadequately housed, 117–21
  nursing, 115, 158, 162, 216; see also
    District nurse

Home (*cont.*)
  and school, conflict between, 51,
    53, 60–6, 189; teachers, 188, 207,
    214
  unattached, 114
  the unmarried, 121–6
Homes
  family group, 130, 140
  grouped cottage, 130, 140
  large, 130, 140
  short-stay, 207
Homosexuality, 96–7
Horder, Lord, 7, 8, 111
Household, 23, 25, 38, 107–8, 165
Housing, Ministry of, and problem
  families, 146
Howells, G. *et al.*, 27
Huxley, A., *Proper Studies*, 56
Hytten, F. E., Yorston, J. C. & Thomson, A. M., 157

Illegitimate child, National Insurance
  Act Allowance, 138
Illingworth, R. S., 44–5, 196; *The
  Normal Child*, 91
Illsley, R., 123
Illustrated London News, 42, 201
Incest, 43, 44, 83, 102
Ineducable child, 190, 195, 197
  appeal to Ministry, 186
  ascertainment, 185, 193
  exclusion, 182, 184
Infant life protection, 138
Ingleby Committee, 83, 148
Institutionalisation, 193, 204
Invalid Children's Aid Association, 217

James, William, *Principles of Psychology*, 18, 47
Jeffreys, M. V. C., *Glaucon*, 66
Journal of Clinical Endocrinology, 14 n.
Journal of Hygiene, 117
Journal of Mental Science, 193
Journal of Pediatrics, 198, 202
Journal of the Royal Sanitary Institute,
  155
Juvenile courts, 76–83

Kahan, V. L. & Fish, J. R., 102
Kanner, K., 198
Kemp, T., 204
Kent, N. & Russell Davies, D., 65 n.

Kirman, B. H., 193
Korsch, B., Fraad, L. & Barnett, H. L.,
  198

Lambert, D. P., 151
Lancet, 121, 149, 153 n., 154, 161, 195
Laws, 29, 30
Lee, J. A., 190
Lennox, W. G., 202
Levy, J. H., 210
Lewis, D. G., 174 n.
Lewis, H., *Deprived Children*, 148
Lightwood, R., Brimblecombe, F. S.
  W., Reinhold, J. D. L., Burnard,
  E. D. & Davis, J. A., 161
Listener, The, 110, 179
Local authority
  adoptions, 126, 128, 129
  assumption of parental rights, 141
  boarding-out, 139
  care of children co-ordinating committee, 146
  Children Act, 138, 139
  Children and Young Persons (Amendment) Act (1952), 142
  children 'Beyond Control', 82
  children's committee, 139; a 'fit
    person', 79
  domiciliary care of premature infants,
    162
  duty to receive children into care,
    138, 139
  and family service unit, 148
  housing, 117
  housing and fireguards, 120
  occasional care of children under
    school age, 138
  parks and playgrounds, 50
  services, proposed expansion of, for
    mental disorder, 194
  teachers of the blind, 214
Local Education authority
  attendance at school, 165–6
  boarding school, 166, 167
  child guidance, 106
  direct grant school, 167, 181
  duty to examine and ascertain handicapped child, 186, 193, 207
  duty to provide a place of education,
    165–6
  duty to provide special educational
    treatment, 207

Local Education Authority (*cont.*)
educationally subnormal, 184–5
employment of children bye-laws, 168
free places, 181
function, 169
general practitioners and inspection sessions, 183
handicapped children, 184–9
hospital school, 188
ineducable, exclusion of, 182, 184
interchange of information with general practitioner, 183
and juvenile court, 77
medical inspection, 52–3, 190
nursery schools, 137
nutrition clinic, 191
problems, 170–3
reserved places, 181
residential education, 138
school health service and private schools, 183; treatment, 183–4
school punishments, 73, 74
subnormal child, 175
transport, 166
visiting teacher, 188
Local Government Finance (H.M.S.O.), 169
Local Health Authority
child guidance, 106
contraceptive advice, 111
day nurseries, 137, 163
and general practitioners, 152
home help, 115, 162
home nursing, 216
maternity and child welfare services, 152
mental health visitor, 207
Nurseries and Child Minders Regulation Act (1948), 137
occupation centre, 186–8
provision for ineducable, 195
Local Housing Authorities and incompetent and problem families, 145
Local Welfare Authority
boarding out, 138, 139
care of children on licence from an approved school, 80
children in care, 'after-care' of, 140
infant life protection, 138

residential nurseries, 140
'short-stay accommodation', 116
Logan, W. P. D., 153
Lost child, *see* Abandoned child
Loneliness, 48
Lunacy acts, 139

MacCarthy, D., Douglas, J. W. B. & Mogford, C., 41
McCoull, G. & Slupinski, L., 205
McKinnon Wood, R., 170
Mackintosh, J. M., *Housing and Family Life*, 117
McLaughlin, M. E., 164
MacMahon, J. F., 187–8
McNeil, C., 156
Magidoff, R., *Yehudi Menuhin*, 87
Magistrates' Association, 142
Maintenance of children, 133–4
Maladjusted Children, Report of the Committee on, 34, 86, 106
Maladjusted children, special classes for, 102
Marriage, 36–9, 101, 132, 180
Marriage and Divorce, Report of the Royal Commission on, 133
Marriage Guidance Council, 131
Marris, P., *Widows and their Families*, 136 n.
Maternity and child welfare services, 137, 150–62
Maternity benefits, 159
Maternity in Great Britain, 153, 154
Mead, M. (ed.), *Cultural Patterns and Technical change*, 41, 42; *New Lives for Old*, 63
Medical attention, 'proper' and minorities, 87
Medical examination
education authority, 52–3; records at juvenile court, 77
L.C.C. child welfare services, 152; L.C.C. schools, 156
remand home, 82
Medical inspection, 183
day nursery, 164
dental, 183
personal hygiene, 183
Medical Inspection and Feeding of Children, Report of the Interdepartmental Committee on, 52

Medical Officer, 103, 106, 115, 121, 122, 123, 145, 148, 151, 176
Medical officer of health, 7, 12, 140, 146, 158
Medical provision for schools, 182–191
Medical Women's Federation, 164
Mental defect, 99, 192–210
  certifications, 195
  among unmarried mothers, 123
  voluntary admission, 195
  see also Handicapped child; Ineducable child; Subnormal child
Mental Deficiency Acts, 139
Mental Health Visitor, 207
Mental Illness and Mental Deficiency, Report of the Royal Commission, 194
Midwives (Local Authority) and hospital co-operation, 161
Miller, F. J. W., 155
Ministry of Health Memorandum on the Prevention and Alleviation of Deafness, 214
Minorities and their children, 87
Moncrieff, A., 155, 190; *Child Health and the State*, 129, 156
Moncrieff, A. & Thomson, W. A. R. (eds.), *Child Health*, 150, 175
Montessori, M., 54, 58–9, 61, 63
Moral danger, 82
Mores, 29, 30, 33
Morris, J. M. & Heady, J. A., 153–4
Mother and baby homes, 124
Mothers
  attitudes to pregnancy, 38–9
  and corporal punishment, 72
  and divorce, 133
  and the handicapped child, 186, 196–203, 207–9, 211
  and the health visitor, 158
  inadequate mothers, 131, 144
  maternity benefits, 159–60
  motherhood education, 143, 151, 156–7
  unmarried, 29, 32, 90, 121–6, 154
  and welfare services, 152–3
Moving from the Slums, 146
Myerson, L., 'A Psychology of Impaired Hearing', 213, 215–16

Naish, C., 155
National Assistance, 13, 136

National Assistance Act, 213
National Assistance Board, 216
National Association of Mental Health, 106 n.
National Birth Control Council, 111
National Health Service Act, 13, 152
National Institute of the Deaf, 217
National Insurance Act
  adoption allowance, 138
  allowance for abandoned child, 138
  allowance for child of divorced parents, 138
  illegitimate child allowance, 138
  orphan child allowance, 138
National Society for the Prevention of Cruelty to Children, 142
Neglect, 82, 141, 143–4, 200–1
Neonatal mortality, 153
Newsholme, A., *Medicine and the State*, 190
New Statesman, 116 n.
Nunn, Sir P., *Education: Its Data and First Principles*, 47, 59
Nurseries and Child Minders Regulation Act (1948), 137
Nursery class, 53, 163
Nursery, residential, 140, 193, 211
Nursery school, 47, 53, 54, 55, 137, 138, 163, 165, 171
Nutrition clinic, 191

Observer, 178
Occupation centre, 186–8, 199, 207
O'Connor, N. & Tizard, J., *The Social Problem of Mental Deficiency*, 197, 205
Oliver, J. N., 176
Orphan Child Allowance, 138
Overcrowding, 108, 109, 116, 117–21

Parent
  duty to provide an education, 165, 166
  unable to exercise, or not exercising, proper care, 82, 138, 139
Parental rights, assumption of by local authority, 141
Parents
  and blind child, 210–14
  and deaf child, 214–17
  and handicapped children, 195–217
  and school medical inspection, 183

Parents' associations, 207–10
Parents' Magazine, 34
Parsons, Sir L., 150
Paul, B. D. (ed.), *Health, Culture and Community*, 19, 27
Pedley, R., *Comprehensive Education*, 177
Physical Deterioration, Report of the Interdepartmental Committee on, 52
Physically handicapped and play therapy, 104
Pinchbeck, I., 125
Pinsent, R. J. F. H.,. *An Approach to General Practice*, 21, 84–5
Play, 46–51, 52
  therapy, 104–6
Pond, D. A. & Bidwell, B., 203
Population, Royal Commission on, Papers of, 111–12
  Report of the Royal Commission on, 155
Prasad, K., 'Ramu the Wolf Boy of Lucknow', 201
Priestley, J. B., *The Neglected Child in the Family*, 141
Prison, 81
Probation
  hostels, 78
  officer, 77, 78, 79, 82, 131
  order, 78
  training homes, 79
Problem families, *see* Family, problem
Prohibitions, 25
Public Health, 7, 26, 29, 96; Act (1936), 138
Public Health, 155
Punishment
  its characteristics, 68–71
  by parents, 71–3
  and responsibility, 67–8, 77
  by society, 75–83
  by teachers, 73–5
  and welfare, 67, 78

Queen's Institute of District Nursing, 160
Querido, A., 145, 193–4

Rathbone, E., 110
Reading Ability, 179
Reception centre, 139

Rehabilitation Literature (1950–5), 207
Religious instruction at school, 166, 167
Remand
  centre, 82
  home, 82
Repond, A., 'Reactions and Attitudes of Families towards their Physically and Mentally Handicapped Children', 200, 216
Research in Public Health, 15
Rewards and Punishments, 73
Rickman, J., 13, 84
Robinson, J. B. Perry, *Report for the National Deaf Children's Society on the Care of the Deaf*, 214 n.
Royal Medico-Psychological Association, *In-Patient Accommodation for Child and Psychiatric Patients*, 104 n.
Royal National Institute for the Blind, 213
Rowntree, B. S. & Lavers, G. R., *English Life and Leisure*, 32
Rules, 25

Saville, P. R., 95
Schonell, F. E., *Educating Spastic Children*, 188
Schools
  aided, 169
  assisted, 182
  attendance, 165–6
  backward classes, 185
  boarding, 166, 167
  comprehensive, 176–7
  controlled, 169
  direct grant, 167, 181
  educationally subnormal, 185
  'finisher', 180
  grammar, 173, 175, 176, 178, 181
  health service, 156, 182–91
  and home, conflict between, 51, 53, 60–5
  hospital, 188
  independent, 167, 182
  maintained, 169
  meals service, 53
  medical provision, 182–91
  nursery, *see* Nursery school
  opportunity classes, 185
  preparatory, 171
  primary, 165–73, 181

Schools (*cont.*)
  private, 171; local authority school
    health service, 183
  progressive, 39, 66
  public, 171, 172, 182
  religious instruction, 166
  residential education, 166, 167, 188–
    9
  secondary, 170, 171, 173, 181
  secondary modern, 173, 176, 177–
    81
  special agreement, 170
  special, medical inspection, 183,
    197 n.
  technical, 173, 175, 176, 178, 181
  unsuitable closure of, 182
Schools for mothers, 150
Scott, J. A., 149
Service education grants, 167
Selye, H., 'The Physiology and Patho-
  logy of Exposure to Stress,' 14 n.
Sexual irregularities in children, 100–2
  see also Incest
Sexual offences against children, 82, 88
  see also Incest
Shanty Town, 50
Shaw-Stewart, P., 56 n.
Sheridan, M. D., 143
Sick child at home, 160–2
Sigarist, H. E., *Medicine and Human
  Welfare*, 89 n.
Simmons, O. G., 'The Clinical Team
  in a Chilean Health Center', 18–
  19
Simon, B., *Intelligence Testing and the
  Comprehensive School*, 174
Smellie, J. M., 160
Social factors in classification of handi-
  cap, 184, 194, 197, 205
Social medicine, 7
Social pressures, 10–17, 39
  and the deprived child, 43
  of the home, 40–5
  of the neighbourhood, 46–51
  of the school, 51–9
Social Service Quarterly, 36
Social Work, 50
Soddy, K., 'Mental Health and the
  Upbringing of Small Children',
  62
Soldiers', Sailors' and Airmen's Family
  Association, 137

Special Educational Treatment, 184, 185
Special reception centre, 82
Spence, Sir James, 18; Spence, Sir J. *et
  al.*, *A Thousand Families in New-
  castle Upon Tyne*, 118, 158
Sperber, Manès, 10
Spock, B., *Baby and Child Care*, 34
Standards of Reading (1948–56), 179
Subnormal child, 175, 176, 184, 185,
  192
  see also Educationally subnormal;
    Ineducable child; Handicapped
    child; Mental defect
Supervision order, 79, 82
Swinscow, D., 120 n.

Tapsfield, J. S., 87
Tavistock Clinic, 94–6
Teachers
  of the blind, 214
  unsuitable, disqualification of, 182
  visiting, 188, 207, 214
Therapeutic relationship, 96–102, 104
  avoidance, 90
  common sense, 90
  limits, 91–4
Times, The, 48, 56, 120 n., 147
Times Educational Supplement, The, 50,
  170, 172, 174, 177
Titmuss, R. M., 110

Valentine, C. W., *The Psychology of
  Early Childhood*, 47
Vaughan, W. T., 'A Frame of Re-
  ference for Family Research in
  Problems of Medical Care', 15
Vernon, P. E. (ed.), *Secondary School
  Selection*, 173
Virchow, R., *Die Medizinische Reform*,
  89

Waller, H., 155
Ward, J. C., *Children out of School*,
  48
Wards of court, 135–6
Watkins, A. G., 161
Way of life, 22, 24, 25, 28, 35, 176
  objective components, 29
  local norms, 31, 32
  subjective components, 29, 88
White-Franklin, A., 195
Widower, 134–5

Widows, 108, 109, 134–5

Widows' cash benefits, 136

Williams, W. M., *The Sociology of an English Village*, 114

Wilkins, E. H., *Medical Inspection of School Children*, 190

Wofinden, R. C., 145

Wolf-boys, 200–1

Woolff, H. G., *Stress and Disease*, 14 n.

Wright, C. H., 148

Wright, G. P. & Wright, H. P., 117

Young, M. & Willmott, P., *Family and Kinship in East London*, 35, 113